Remo Rittiner: Yoga Therapy For Health and Healing

Yoga Therapy For Health and Healing
Yoga Practice for Health and Clarity

Remo Rittiner

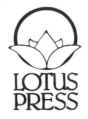

LOTUS
PRESS

Twin Lakes, WI

First published in Germany 2011 by Verlag Via Nova

First US Edition published by Lotus Press, 2013

2nd printing, 2014

Translated from the original German by Amanda Johnston

WARNING

This book is not intended as an alternative to personal, professional yoga instruction. If you have any concerns about your current level of health or fitness then you should consult your doctor before partaking in any new exercise programme. Neither the author nor the publisher accept any responsibility for injury that may occur from use of this material.

Printed in the United States of America

ISBN: 978-0-9409-8514-8

formerly published by Bookshaker under ISBN: 978-1-907498-82-4

Library of Congress Control Number: 2013945102

Printed In USA

Published by:

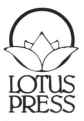

Lotus Press
P.O. Box 325
Twin Lakes, WI 53181 USA
800-824-6396 (toll free order phone)
262-889-8561 (office phone)
262-889-2461 (office fax)
www.lotuspress.com (website)
lotuspress@lotuspress.com (email)

I dedicate this book to my children,
Anand and Anjali

Acknowledgements

My sincerest thanks to

A. Mohan and R. Sriram, who passed on to me my most valuable knowledge about the yoga tradition from T. Krishnamacharya.

Gary Kraftsow and John Kepner from the USA, who have supported me in my yoga teaching.

Uta Naumer-Hotz and Alexander Hotz from Constance for writing the invaluable anatomy texts and for cooperating with me on this book.

Dr. Chandrakant Pawar from India and Dr. John Switzer from Germany, who wrote the Ayurveda recommendations for chronic conditions.

Klaus König from BDY and Karin Ueckert, who enhanced both the exercise programme and the anatomy text with their suggestions. All photo models from the yoga therapy training group, who were willing to participate in the yoga programme on a regular basis.

Kathrin Rick for the linguistic review of the manuscripts and Eveline Keller, who helped to integrate the texts. The Fuchs photography studio in Zurich and photographer Nicole Blatter for the superb photographs.

Dr. Rüdiger Dahlke for the foreword and his much appreciated support. Werner Vogel from Via Nova publishing for his confidence and generous support for the book.

All yoga students and yoga therapists, who accompany me on the path of yoga.

Amanda Johnston of D.Code Translations in the UK, who translated the book from its original German into English.

Susan Gilbert from Florida for the first 10 antomical illustrations in the book.

Contents

Foreword

I was delighted about the creation of this book and to be asked to write the foreword, as I have known the author for a long time and value his expertise but above all his calm and composure. In my Swiss dental further training seminars, he has demonstrated in a most impressive way how well yoga can be used as therapy. He has also offered valuable advice regarding posture, even for people who are constantly working under great stress. Remo Rittiner has enriched these medical advanced training seminars time and again, not only through his therapeutic interventions in which he selects the correct exercises for damage that has already occurred, but also in the sense of preventative suggestions from his treasure chest of yoga asanas. Even at a personal level, unfortunately – or rather, fortunately – I have had the opportunity to put Remo's suggestions for my own back problems into practice. Not only did these exercises help but they were fun too. This is one of his open secrets in the seminars – how enjoyable yoga can be. I believe that he has also managed to put across the sensual and joyful commitment to this ancient art in his book – as well as between its lines. Unless something is enjoyable it will be no help in the long run – and this is also true of practices in the realm of physical exercise and therapies. His dedicated texts make it clear time and again how yoga, even when it is presented in a topic-based and problem-orientated way, as it is here, has a great deal more to offer than just postural and physical exercise. The author's understanding and communication of the belief that an inner attitude corresponds with every external posture on which it

ultimately depends has forged our long cooperation in the seminars. The body is considered to be of great importance but only as the springboard to a free and open mind. Therefore, it is obviously preferable for the mind to be accommodated in a free, powerful and mobile body. "How are you?" we ask innocently. Actually, we can read from a person's stance how they are and how their life is – perhaps fixed and secure or balanced and fluid. We can even tell whether what they say is true and what they may be facing in life. How they are shows how they proceed, how they progress, how they advance in life and how they are doing with it, in addition to whether they will continue to be all right or whether they were even all right in the first place. Their posture and attitude are very revealing. Let's look at one of the many wonderful chapters of this book in a little more detail – the one concerning feet. These are accorded little space in many yoga books, yet they are the basis of our life – our roots – and they are given the importance they deserve in this book. Thus, to improve your state through the yoga postures described and shown in pictures, is also to benefit from the positive effect this has on your life, in feeling more grounded and even grounding your attitudes. In the corresponding exercises, the book deals with all the significant areas of a person, based on a sound anatomical foundation, so that it is possible to uplift all aspects of yourself and to align them with the ideal, to become a more sincere and harmonious person inside. Physical posture will of course convey this externally and everyone else will notice it. The difference between a person who practises yoga in the spirit of this book and a bodybuilder could not be greater. The yoga student shapes his or her body in the process but also advances the mind, which is at the core of everything. A bodybuilder would be unlikely to be able to explain the nature of a well-formed mind. We can therefore improve the inner attitude through the outer – ideally using the exercises presented here. In this respect, each yoga posture is inspired by the hope that the inner follows the outer.

If someone sits in the Lotus position and thereby imitates Buddha, this could be viewed as presumptuous for they are assuming a position which can in no way correspond to their inner state. However, their hope is to aspire to exactly that. They therefore sit in this position but they are focused on the mind. Bodybuilding too can of course operate in this conscious way. This attitude can essentially be applied way beyond the practice of yoga and could even apply to a visit to the hair salon. A new hairstyle also brings new form, but only at an outer level. However, the next stage would be to apply this form internally too. Or put more simply, twiddling locks of your hair does not automatically make you alluring; the inner attitude and the radiance of being seductive must first be cultivated.

"Yoga" comes from the word yoke, the device that brings together the strength of two oxen into one. It originally meant uniting and combining body and mind, form and content. The exercises in this book are eminently suitable for becoming one with your body by gaining awareness of the topics associated with every part of the physique. This is a wonderful way to grow and mature, by integrating each theme with your own body. And of course all archetypally important principles relate to their specific areas of the body.

Yoga is clearly a holistic system of self-realisation. This would not be a therapy book if it did not also include a section for those requiring repair or correction. In the form in which it is being taught here, yoga can help alleviate problems in many areas. However, it can also support the success of other therapies. Hence, there is a section dedicated to major symptoms particularly well served by yoga therapy.

However, the most fascinating aspect of this book remains the author himself, Remo Rittiner. I have never known him to speak from prepared texts, not even when he gave his first talk in front of 180 doctors. But he has never come across as unprepared; he is not only teaching yoga, but he is living in the moment – and therefore the moment serves him and always delivers him the right words. When you know him longer you can have the feeling that he is yoga. Remo can therefore teach and convey yoga without any sense of ambition or stress. This books shows he can write in this way too.

Ruediger Dahlke, April 2009

(www.dahlke.at)

Introduction to Ayur yoga therapy

"The small hole in her heart has fused together again by itself. Your little daughter, Anjali, is completely healthy."

This is what a doctor told me, after I had begun to write *Yoga Therapy For Health and Healing*. As confident as I was prior to the positive news, I cannot help but feel extremely grateful. During my many years of work as a yoga therapist, I have had great trust in a person's self-healing power. Yoga is the connection with the universal power of self-healing, which we can see in nature and in all beings. The Ayur yoga therapy presented in this book is centred on the basic principles of the yoga tradition of Krishnamacharya, the knowledge of Ayurveda and the latest anatomical information. It brings together the traditional empirical sciences of yoga and Ayurveda with the modern science of functional anatomy and muscular function therapy. In the holistic view of the person, Ayur yoga therapy recognises the interaction and dynamics between body, breathing, mind, nutrition and way of life, and their effect on the state of our health. The person and their resources are at the forefront of yoga therapy. It is therefore a case of recognising the circumstances, behaviour and habits that have brought the state of health out of balance. In essence, it is less to do with symptoms and illnesses, but more about the causes that have led to the complaint.

Back pain, for example, often has multiple causes, for example, muscular tension in the groin, abdomen and hips, which has a negative effect on abdominal breathing. This reduces the effectiveness of the dia-phragm, connected to the pericardium. The abdomen may be bloated, the digestion sluggish and the bowel movements irregular. Mental pressures such as stress, existential fears or repressed feelings may also be causes of back problems.

The widely-held view that it is sensible to strengthen the abdomen when there is back pain, is counter-productive in many cases and may, for example, further increase disc problems. It is only when we look at the person as a whole that it is possible to recognise the various causes of their symptoms, such as back problems. This enables us to successfully treat the causes of the complaint using the myriad resources of yoga. Yoga practice is individually adapted to the person – based on their age, state of health and life circumstances. Following a detailed initial discussion and case history, an individual yoga programme is compiled that can be worked on regularly at home.

Practising yoga independently gives you the chance to help yourself. Accepting our complaints opens up space for self-reflection and new ways of dealing with them to support our capacities for self-healing. An important point in teaching yoga is to create the preconditions for a calm and clear mind. Through varied exercises for the body, the breath and the mind, yoga therapy offers us excellent opportunities to regain peace and clarity. In this way we can more clearly perceive our relationship to ourselves and our environment, reflect on our behaviour and independently answer important questions in our lives.

In my work as a yoga therapist, I am always fascinated to observe how people find the answers within themselves when their mind is calm. Connection with a clear mind opens up incredible opportunities for healing and transformation at all levels of being – at physical, emotional and mental levels.

Experiencing the manifold healing effects of yoga therapy inspires me anew with each person. My own practical experience tells me that yoga therapy can be helpful for back pain, neck tension, knee problems, high blood pressure, migraine, digestive complaints, constipation, asthma, sleep issues, PMS syndrome, cancer, AIDS, overcoming stress, grieving, overweight, anxiety, depression, bullying, eating disorders, preparing for pregnancy, burnout syndrome, life crises, relationship difficulties and many chronic illnesses.

I would like to open the door to Ayur yoga therapy for you. I want to inspire you to experience it for yourself and to find the potential for your self-healing capacity. This book gives you the foundations of yoga therapy and various yoga programmes, and a chance to use them and experience their effects.

The objectives of *Yoga Therapy For Health and Healing* are as follows:

- To provide you with the most important foundations for effective yoga practice

- To combine yoga with the most up-to-date knowledge of anatomy

- To familiarise you with the healing potential of yoga therapy

- To show you many effective yoga exercises that you can do yourself

- To pave the way for you to practise yoga independently using targeted programmes, which may be helpful for certain complaints

- To motivate you to practise yoga regularly and with variety

- To introduce you to a meditation technique which can bring holistic health and clarity

- To inspire you to integrate the wisdom of yoga into your life

Chapter One tells you about the foundations for successful, independent practice of the yoga programme. The success of your yoga practice depends on many factors, such as clear understanding of the exercises, effective practice, self-motivation and the willingness to perform them regularly.

Take time to absorb the first chapter before you start with the exercise programme.

Chapter Two, Structural Yoga Therapy, has generally therapeutic yoga programmes, from healthy feet to a healthy neck. Before each one, read the important information on the functional anatomy and the objective of the yoga programme.

Chapter Three details yoga therapy programmes for chronic complaints. Ayurveda tips provide you with valuable information to encourage and support the capacity for self-healing.

Chapter Four explains important steps for healing and transformation through yoga. Besides this, there are

Instructions for effective yoga meditation, which can assist you with your health and with attaining a clear mind.

Chapter 1: The foundations of yoga therapy

The internal attitude determines the effect

"There now follows an introduction to yoga – *atha yoga anusasanam*" – this is the first yoga sutra of the sage, Patanjali.

Be aware of your inner and outer state at this moment. How does your posture feel? How do you feel within at this moment?

These are two interesting questions that lead you directly into the now and into life. If you ask yourself such questions regularly, your thoughts and actions will alter. In what way will you change?

Before you continue reading, remain within and give yourself time to reflect upon these questions.

Reflection gives us the opportunity to observe our current mental state. According to yoga philosophy, the mind, and everything that is perceptible, possesses three qualities: heaviness, activity and clarity. You will read, perceive and understand this text differently, depending on the dominant characteristic. If you are very active, it is possible that you will skim over these pages. If your mental state is crystal clear, it is likely you find it easy to reflect and that you have insight into important topics. With a tired mind, you will find it difficult to gain such understanding.

With the variety of yoga exercises for the body, breath and mind, it is possible for us to deepen the perception of all three qualities. Mental obstacles such as misconceptions, self-preoccupation, desires, antipathy and anxieties distort our perception of our own internal attitudes and mental states.

Of course, yoga practice will also lead us to encounter the so-called mental barriers, the *kleshas* (causes of suffering).

"Stop exercising! That's not yoga as I teach it." When I said this recently in a yoga class, Peter looked at me astounded. "You're making too much effort with the physical exercises", I told him and saw absolute amazement in his face. Beaming and visibly relieved, he said to the yoga group present that nobody had said such a thing to him in the last 45 years. This statement touched me deeply.

At the level of understanding many people are surely aware that they are stressed and are therefore blocking their life energy (*prana*). We can all find the roots of this widely held misconception of over-exerting yourself in any form in the causes of suffering, the *kleshas*.

For example, imposing difficult yoga exercises on others, the fear of not fulfilling the demands of the teacher or their own demands, reluctance to expose oneself to something unfamiliar, misunderstanding of the laws of nature, or exaggerated attachment to the body – such motives can drive us into a corner time and again, create unwholesome actions (*dukha*) and increase the anguish. From the perspective of yoga, it is all about reducing distress and opening up space for clarity and freedom. The following inner attitudes are helpful for the effectiveness of yoga practice:

- Your intent and objective should be clear

- Practise with joy and lightness

- Do the exercises with relaxed mindfulness

- Practise fondly and respect your own limitations

- Be tolerant with yourself and do not make judgments about yourself

- Be patient with impatience and look forward to small advances

- Be bold in trying new experiences and face the challenge of more difficult exercises

- Keep the effect of the exercise to the fore and not its outer form

- Find your balance between stability and relaxation

- Remain natural and smile when practising

- Feel the strength of your commitment

- Appreciate your efforts and give thanks when completing your yoga practice

Recognising and changing unhealthy physical postures

Your internal attitude will have a considerable effect on your yoga practice. The responsibility is therefore entirely yours. If you emphasise one of the qualities mentioned when practising yoga and in your everyday life, you will be astounded at how effective yoga is. Open up your potential and delight in your success. You can of course consciously promote these internal attitudes in your daily life.

Your posture will always tell you how you are feeling. Our physical stance and movement patterns reflect our emotional and mental state. The varied movement in yoga offer the opportunity to become familiar with our attitudes and movement patterns.

In the various yoga traditions, opinions on the teaching of correct posture and carrying out yoga exercises frequently differ starkly. Often they do not agree with current knowledge of western anatomy. In yoga teaching and in yoga teacher training, many participants speak of their uncertainty about which position is right or wrong.

Terms such as right or wrong can lead us to view things very one-sidedly and dogmatically. An open mind allows different opinions, however, which we will look at in more detail. Based on this objective of achieving the optimum effect with yoga, we can check whether a teaching view is helpful. If we consciously experience the different effects of postures and movements, we are personally in a position to judge what feels good and correct and what we should avoid. Of course, this presupposes openness to always checking our own attitudes and concepts. It requires courage and humility to question qualified people and sometimes to let it go.

As a yoga therapist, I have the opportunity for open exchanges with many who practise yoga and with various yoga and anatomy experts. I I have thus developed my own point of view, which has been proven in practice. As an experienced practitioner, it is always worthwhile looking anew and taking an approach in the spirit of the beginner.

Our posture and movements have a major effect on our well-being and vitality. Imagine someone delivering a PowerPoint presentation on sincerity with a rounded back and hunched shoulders! Would the speaker appear credible or unbelievable?

A naturally upright posture enables the flow of our life energy (*prana*). Have you ever thought how much energy it takes to remain uptight? That rounding the back negatively affects our breathing? The effect that poor posture has on the psyche?

In the following images you will have the opportunity to check your posture from head to toe. In each initial image you will see the posture that is closest to being optimum and natural, from an anatomical perspective. Below it are two typically unhealthy examples. Using the yoga programmes in this book, you will then be able to practise the optimum postures. You should of course integrate these postures into your everyday life. Take the time and be patient, if you are changing the pattern of your posture. You will probably slip back into the old patterns. This already speaks of success and the start of change; for many people are not even aware of their unhealthy posture.

Feet

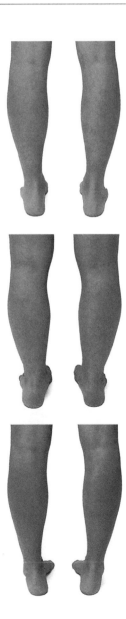

Optimum loading of weight on feet
Even weight on the heels and the front of the foot is important for stable and statically correct posture.

Talipes valgus (skew foot)
Lack of stability and unfavourable load for the joints and toes.

Heavy loading on the outer edge
Lack of stability for the joint of the big toe and overloading of the ligaments.

Alignment of the legs

Optimum orientation of the legs
Stability and anatomically correct loading of weight on the feet. Optimum alignment for the hip, knee and ankle joints. Good transfer of weight to the legs and healthy weight on the knees.

Knock Knees
Instability and risk of arthrosis on the outside of the knee. Incorrect pressure on the feet. Lack of grounding and contact with the ground.

Bandy legs
Instability and risk of arthrosis on the inside of the knees. Unfavourable stress on the hip joints.

Knees

Optimum knee stability
Stability for the knee joint and effective transmission of energy to the legs.

Knees turned inwards
Instability and overloading of the knees. Adverse pressure on the lower back and reduced transfer of energy.

Overstretched knees
Instability. Too much strain on the knees. Risk of damage to the knee (very widespread in yoga circles).

Spine

Optimum alignment of the spine
Even weight on the spine and the discs in the back. Enables space for the organs and for deep breathing. Creates the optimum conditions for the pelvic floor, groin and hip joints. Conveys energy and sincerity at a psychic level.

Severe hyperlordosis (curvature)
Overloading of the small vertebral joints and ligaments in the lower back. Slackens the pelvic floor and encourages lowering of the organs. Reduces the breath by narrowing the lungs.

Lack of alignment in the spine
Places an adverse strain on the discs and encourages rounding of the back. Causes tension in the pelvic floor and shoulder area. Leads to poor breathing and constipation. Gives a feeling of pulling in the back.

Pelvis

Optimum pelvic position
Even weight on the hip joints and spine. Stable centre of the body and even muscle activity.

Tilted pelvis
Unstable posture with pelvic scoliosis. Uneven load on the spine and hip joints. Danger of iliosacral joint blocking. Indication of possible scoliosis.

Protruding pelvis
Unstable posture with uneven load across the whole body. Chronic, asymmetric muscle tension. Sign of scoliosis. Unfavourable for even breathing.

Chest

Optimum chest position

Relaxed muscles in the chest and shoulder area. Facilitates thoracic breathing and creates space in the lungs. Opens up the heart and promotes healthy self-confidence.

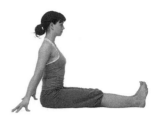

Collapsed chest

Takes up space for deep breathing and for the organs. Leads to muscular tension in the chest area. Decreases the breath in the ribs and chest. May block vertebrae, ribs and joints. Brings out feelings of withdrawal and anxiety.

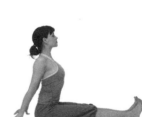

Protruding chest

Causes muscular tension between the shoulder blades and in the upper back. Makes the thoracic spine stiff. Promotes the feeling of arrogance and pride. Gives an appearance of seeming pretentious and overbearing.

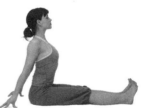

Optimum half spinal twist

Encourages the mobility of the thoracic spine and ribs. Deepens thoracic breathing and expands the chest muscles. Brings stability and is very centring for the mind. Promotes grace and self-respect.

Evasive spinal twist

Instability and less movement in the thoracic spine. The pelvis turns too. Gives the illusion of moving the chest (common movement pattern in yoga circles).

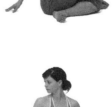

Compressed spinal twist

The spine is not straight and there is a lack of movement in the thoracic spine. Causes tension in the neck and shoulder area. Unhealthy for the discs. The breathing is shallow and superficial. Leads to clumsiness in the body and mind.

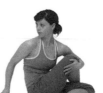

Shoulders

Optimum shoulders

Upright posture and relaxed neck. Ideal shoulder position and good functioning of the shoulder joints. Relaxed shoulders and free breathing. Gives a sense of lightness and has an energising effect.

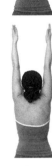

Raised shoulders

Leads to tension in the shoulder and neck area. Unfavourable position for the shoulder joint and can lead to wear.

Hanging shoulders

Causes muscle tension in the chest area. Restricts the breath and prevents deep breathing. Neck tension and strain on the discs. Leads to anxiety and withdrawal into a protective position.

Arms

Optimum arm stability

Stable posture and optimum weight on the joints in the shoulders, elbows and wrists. Effective transmission of energy to the arm and shoulder muscles.

Unstable arms

Poor transfer of energy between the trunk and arms. Overloading of the joints and instability.

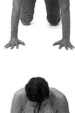

Overstretched arms

Over-extension of the ligaments and elbows. Poor transmission of energy to the arms and trunk muscles. May lead to various elbow and shoulder complaints (common posture pattern in yoga circles).

Neck

Optimum neck position

The weight is spread ideally between the cervical spine and discs. The breath can flow freely and there is no pressure on the air pipes. The shoulder and neck muscles work optimally without being tense.

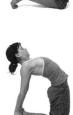

Compressed neck

The discs and the vertebrae of the neck are compressed and under pressure. Breathing is in short bursts. The neck and shoulder muscles are tense.

Overstretched cervical spine

A great deal of strain on the discs in the neck. There tends to be instability in the neck. The throat and shoulder muscles are under tension.

The art of joyful effort

Finding the right degree of effort is the key to making the most of your yoga practice. Expressions such as "You can only be successful if you work hard" are widespread and characteristic of our western, goal-oriented society. From early childhood on, we learn quickly that we receive affection and acknowledgement because of our external achievements. Patanjali, in the sutra 1-14 of Yoga Sutras, tells us

"Success beckons only to those who work intensively and sincerely. The chances for success depend upon the degree of the effort."

In the Yoga Sutras of Patanjali, yoga asanas (postures) are defined as having the qualities of *sthiramsukham asanam*, roughly translated as "stability and ease".

When we practice yoga, it is a holistic exercise of physical and mental awareness. If we use a mind-set of ambition and achievement to force ourselves into a difficult yoga posture, we will be unable to reach the quality of stability and ease. In this case, what we are really doing is not yoga but physical gymnastics. In order to develop a yoga practice that is healthy and healing, it is essential to keep in mind the yogic approach and the holistic effects on the body, breath and mind.

Attentive practice, performed with the right degree of effort, gives us the opportunity to experience all the wonderful benefits of yoga. In yoga practice in which we use brute force to achieve a posture, over-exertion causes the structure to become unstable, the breath to become restricted, and the mind to become tense. If we stay too long in this posture, our physical strength wanes and the balance of our energy system becomes disturbed.

Modern research into strength training has shown that too much physical training causes an overall decrease in muscle strength and weakens the immune system. It is therefore no coincidence that many competitive athletes are often afflicted with colds. Interestingly, in my work as a physical therapist, I have observed that those who undertake very physically demanding yoga practice often have weak and highly contracted muscles. Initially, this surprised me because I had expected that flexible and fit people would be less tense. In order to experience the art of holistic strength training, I encourage you to try the following:

- Stand upright.

- Straighten your right leg and lift it up.

- At the same time, concentrate on the muscles in the front of your right thigh and contract them as much as possible. As you contract the muscles, notice the results of the effort on your breath and emotions. After a short time, let your leg come down.

- Next, do the same exercise as before, but this time, smile as you work hard to lift your leg.

- Now, keep your smile while you are engaging your muscles and look for a sense of relaxation while letting the leg work.

- Try both methods, and see if you notice a difference in the strength of your thigh muscles and the quality of your breath and mind when you smile.

What did you experience during this exercise?

Practising with a relaxed internal attitude helps us to experience joyful effort. Applying this attitude to our yoga practice offers us the sacred gift of holistic well-being. I am often reminded of the looks I have received from avid body builders in the gym during my numerous experiments on strength training machines. They obviously found the light weights I worked with were disproportionate to my size and would have encouraged me to use heavier ones. However, with the yogic attitude and special yoga breathing techniques, I was amazed by how much strength training can accomplish, even with light weights, if the mind is relaxed and the body is not over-exerted.

The art of joyful effort lies in striving sincerely and devotedly in a particular direction without overdoing it. If, for example, this attitude is absent during a stretch, we will not achieve the maximum stretch or increased mobility we seek. Instead, without maintaining these internal qualities, we may over-stretch or even injure ourselves. With all yoga exercises, we can determine whether or not we have succeeded in finding joyful effort by looking for the following characteristics

- Do we feel harmonious?

- Is the flow of our breath smooth and undisturbed?

- Do we feel that the challenge of the exercise is something for which we are prepared?

- Are we experiencing physical and mental development?

- Are we feeling joy and openness?

Adapting yoga practice to your own needs

It is worthwhile practising the art of joyful effort in our daily life as well. Approach it with patience; for many people, exerting less is a completely new way of thinking and acting. Since I have started exerting less in my life, I have been more at ease, more joyful, and more successful. For some of the most successful people in the world, it seems as though they do not exert effort and yet they achieve success none the less.

The personal adaptation of yoga practice to individuals is an important part of the yoga tradition of the Indian Yoga master, T. Krishnamacharya. By closely observing and clarifying a person's needs, it is possible to devise an effective yoga practice. The following factors should play a part:

- Age
- Personality
- Physical and mental constitution
- Condition of health
- Diet
- Lifestyle
- Occupation
- Family relationships
- Spiritual orientation
- Willingness and discipline to practise yoga
- Needs and objectives

In individual yoga teaching, it is possible for an experienced yoga therapist to take account of all these factors. It is thereby possible for an individual to achieve a high degree of quality and effectiveness in practising yoga.

Exercising regularly based on the instructions of a yoga therapist creates favourable conditions for achieving the objectives set. Yoga is increasingly integrated into the daily life, thus opening up the path to physical health and mental clarity. No book on yoga can create these optimum preconditions for you.

Developing yoga practice

Vinyasa Krama is a tried and tested concept from the Indian yoga tradition of T. Krishnamacharya, which is being successfully applied throughout the world by many successful yoga teachers. *Vinyasa Krama* means "intelligent steps in stages".

Setting objectives, preparation, introduction and balance are all elements of a yoga programme. The intent and setting of objectives should be realistic. The practice should help us reach goals in small stages. In my work as a yoga therapist, I place great importance on practising with a clear objective and constantly checking whether these aims suit the circumstances.

Many people come into yoga therapy because of health problems such as back pain. Their foremost consideration is self-healing. We stimulate the powers of self-healing via gentle physical and breathing exercises as well as relaxation and reflection. Once the backache has gone we must strengthen the back. Such preventative measures promote good health on a lasting basis. As soon as the back is strengthened, we ultimately want to find out which mental qualities would be helpful in the current situation. Now breath, self-reflection and meditation are central to the practice.

Many people who come into yoga therapy have a need to find their own answer to important life questions. The areas of health, self-healing and spiritual development are often helpful. The holistic effects of yoga exercise, frequently addresses many levels of the person.

The three steps: intent, breath and movement

The intent of the exercise should be clear. In the practice part of this book, under "Effect", you can see what the intent is and where the focus of this exercise lies. If, when exercising, you set several focal points all at once, there is the risk of over-extending yourself and reducing the effect. However, by concentrating your attention in a very targeted way, you will further increase the positive effects of the exercises. Before you carry out a movement you must get in touch with your breathing. This brings you into the now and connects you with the energy of the breath. You undertake the intended exercise whilst keeping your attention with the breath. You can apply this model to many situations in life. It works beautifully if you carry out activities in a more conscious way.

For example, if you wish to express an opinion to somebody, it is very helpful to be clear about your own intent. If you then become conscious of your breathing, there is a very good chance that you will carry out your actions more carefully. Try it yourself today! And when you experience a feeling of tension in future life situations, then remember this experience.

Preparation, introduction and balance

To begin with, we select exercise that fit in with the practice. The preparatory exercises are already linked to the objectives. Start with gentle, simple, mobilising exercises; your body will be grateful to you if you do not start straight away with the headstand or salute to the sun.

Be aware of your current condition. Respect this during further practice. You progress slowly through the exercises in small stages until you manage a main exercise. For example, you can commence with gentle forward bends before ending with a challenging static forward bend in which you can stay while sitting.

The dynamic exercise in yoga is an ideal preparation for being able to remain longer in difficult positions. Modern yoga teaching is increasingly about pushing through. Tension may result from doing strenuous exercises, especially where there is over-exertion. It is therefore sensible to integrate balancing exercises into your programme.

Pay attention to the transitions between the exercises. For example, going from standing exercises directly into lying on the back, may cause a person with low blood pressure to feel faint. Or if you climb straight into a car after mediation, the pleasant condition of inner floating could threaten your safety. The ideal creation of a practice, the so-called *Vinyasa Krama*, is an art and science in itself.

Adaptations of the postures and exercises

In modern yoga practice, the exercises are increasingly being adapted to the needs and preconditions of Westerners. Acrobatic contortions or difficult back bends are practised with more care or not at all. It has also become clear to many people that the European physique is different to the Indian. However, there are also followers of yoga trends who do not wish to know about this. With the argument that it is "traditional yoga", yoga exercises are carried out which have not been adapted to the capabilities of the people practising them. In my work as a yoga therapist I often meet people who have sustained injuries through yoga. We must therefore look closely at which exercises are reasonable for us and which ones may be damaging. The most up-to-date exercise teaching with the latest anatomical knowledge may be helpful to us in the choice and instruction of the exercises. In this way, the ancient science of yoga can be sensibly combined with the Western anatomy.

Techniques for adapting the exercises

There are various options for adapting the postures and movements. If it is not possible for you to carry out the entire movement given or assume the final posture, simply go as far into the movement or position as your body allows. Pay attention to your feelings and accept your limits. If an exercise causes pain, this is a warning signal from your body. In future, you should only carry out this movement up to the point where it does not hurt. By reducing the intensity of a strengthening or stretching move and then increasing it in stages, you will be safer and will exercise more efficiently. Your body will be grateful to you for your sympathetic way of moving. Observe the wisdom of your body, which tells you exactly what will do it good and what will not. We will be richly rewarded for careful, gentle and sincere movements.

Practice with the wisdom of the body

To give you the opportunity to experience the wisdom of the body itself, I invite you to try the following exercise. Come on to your back, bend your knees and bring your feet to the floor. Hold on to the back of your right thigh with both hands.

Exhaling, pull your leg towards the body allowing the foot to lift off of the floor and the knee to bend slightly. You will probably feel a stretch in the muscles at the back of the thigh. Notice the sensation while you firmly hold the leg toward you. Now, reduce the effort by slightly bending the leg to let the thigh move a little more toward the body. Be aware of what you experience in the back of the right thigh. With your next exhalation, gently let the leg move even closer to the body so a slight stretching sensation remains in the back of the right leg but without experiencing a strong pull. Keep the leg in the same position when inhaling. During the next exhalation, carefully pull the leg towards you again. Take two or three minutes to go, step by step (*Vinyasa Krama*) more deeply into the exercise. After you finish, reflect on what your body has taught you. We often achieve more if we want less.

This concept of small steps (micro-movements) in our attitudes toward stretching can also be used in strengthening exercises to find a deeper experience. This approach to exercise becomes incredibly important when we work with yoga breathing practices (*Pranayama*).

The body is grateful when we give it space and time to experience something new; this is also true for our mind. A secret of life, which I have been able to find through yoga exercises, is to open to this space. If you experience this openness or expansiveness in your postures, you are working with the very essence of yoga. Listen to your breath when you practise. The flow of the breath will become more regular and extended if we are in balance. If you feel over-exerted in a posture or during a practice, allow yourself to rest, then wait until your breath flows evenly again before continuing. You can simplify exercises by, for example, slightly bending the knees in a standing forward bend if your hamstrings are tight. Also, observe the speed at which you move in exercises, and notice if the tempo matches your current energy level or the level of energy you are trying to achieve, i.e. are you trying to find a calm state of mind by jumping quickly from posture to posture or moving slowly and thoughtfully between postures? Never let anyone force a breathing rhythm that does not work for you.

It is generally advisable to avoid hasty movements in your yoga practice. They put you at risk of injury, disturb the breath, and prevent the mind from becoming calm. If you are looking for a more challenging physical practice, you can increase the intensity by either moving more slowly or simply slowing down the flow of the breath. Using awareness and attention as your guide, you will find that your body clearly indicates when it is ready for more difficult postures. Do not let yourself be guided by the desire to achieve external goals or measure up to an ideal form of a posture defined by someone else.

In the practice of yoga, we are more concerned with the quality of the effect of the practice rather than an arbitrary measure of achievement. The external form of the posture is not the primary goal. However, our ego will often try to divert us again and again from the more essential but less obvious objectives. When we practice with awareness, we will repeatedly be led deeper into the moment. Discover the endless wisdom of your body and mind by adapting yoga practices to your own needs.

A yogi is a person who meets changing circumstances with an open heart and who behaves appropriately in each situation. The ability to adapt to life is a reflection of open consciousness.

The healing power of yoga breathing techniques

The breath is the gateway to physical health and self-healing. A gentle breath leads you direct into the stillness of being. Calming the movement of the mind is the classic yoga definition by Patanjali, meaning 'it breathes'.

Have you ever wondered about the energy we create with the breath?

Focus inward for a while. Pay attention to your breath. Listen to it. Now ask yourself what energy breathing directs? Give space to this question and receive the answer. News from the inner world is free and very valuable. The science of the breath is called *Pranayama* in yoga. This Sanskrit (Indian language of scholars) expression can be translated as "expansion of the breath". In many books on yoga it is translated as "controlling the breath". My own experience tells me it is less about control and much more about spiritual opening, which enables the breath to expand. When you pay attention to breathing it changes in quality.

This passive form of *Pranayama* is an important part of Vipassana meditation (Buddhist meditation technique) and other forms of meditation. The orientation of the mind to the breath leads us into a meditative state. Breathing is the most important nourishment in our lives and its quality has a considerable influence on our life energy. It is no coincidence that in today's world many people breathe shallowly and irregularly. It has probably already occurred to you how negatively physical indisposition affects our breathing.

You can discover a great deal about your current mental condition through the quality of your breathing. In yoga, we change our breathing pattern consciously to achieve physical and mental balance. In *Pranayama* there are numerous breathing techniques which you can learn best with an experienced yoga teacher. The breath is so powerful that we can also damage our health with it. I remember one of my first intensive yoga courses, in which the yoga teacher carried out very intensive breathing exercises with long pauses in the breath. Many participants had strong reactions such as an inability to concentrate and sleep problems. As with physical exercises, with *Pranayama*, its adaptation to people should be of the utmost importance.

Extend the breath by breathing in the throat

One of the most effective breathing techniques in yoga is breathing with the throat, which is sometimes known as 'throat breathing', or, in Sanskrit as *Ujjayi* (pronounced "udschai"). It is an effective technique to extend and refine the breath. We contract the glottis in the larynx. This produces a sound which we can hear. We receive feedback via this sound as to whether our breath is long and even. We can use this technique for all physical exercises and it helps us carry out movements more harmoniously.

Breathing through the throat optimises the extension and energising effect of physical exercise. It encourages concentration and mindfulness.

Technique for throat breathing

Assume an upright sitting position. Make a 'ha' sound with your throat, as though you were trying to breathe on a frozen car window. Open your mouth when doing this. After a few repetitions, close the mouth and repeat the 'ha' sound from the throat several times. You should now hear the fricative sound of air in the throat. Vary the 'ha' sound by changing its intensity. To begin with, most people have to accustom themselves to throat breathing but once you have learned this technique, you will find it difficult not to do it. Practice throat breathing initially exhaling. After a while you can also practice throat breathing inhaling. Avoid forcing it out. The sound should be at such a level that the person sitting next to you in a yoga class, or to whom you are introducing yourself, can hardly hear it. As it is about the refinement of your breathing, your sounds should not cause any physical or mental tension. Remember the proviso of joyful effort.

The effects of "throat breathing"

- Increases the breathing volume
- Strengthens and expands the lungs
- Cleans the larynx and expectorates
- Improves circulation in the throat
- Increases the intake of oxygen and the expulsion of carbon dioxide
- Purging and alkalising effect
- Stimulates the digestion and excretory organs
- More effective strengthening and stretching of the body
- Releases muscular and emotional tension
- Increases concentration and wellbeing
- Stimulates endorphins
- Connects with divine energy

You should not practise throat breathing if you have high blood pressure, heart complaints, are going through the menopause and hot flushes or are suffering from severe asthma. If you are unsure, ask your yoga therapy expert and consult a doctor.

Breathing leads movement

In the physical exercises of yoga, we lead movement using throat breathing. Breathing encompasses movement. For example, when you inhale and lift the arms, then you exhale and lower the arms. This ensures mindfulness and optimum coordination of breath and movement. You also guard against quick, hasty movements that can lead to injury.

As we direct the attention to the chest when we breathe in, the inhalation supports the stretching of the thoracic spine. When we gently draw in the lower abdominal as we exhale, this extends the lower back and also strengthens the abdominal muscles. Even if you have learned another breathing technique for yoga exercises, I would recommend trying out this technique of inhalation and exhalation during exercises. Raise and lower your arms a few times using this technique. Now repeat the raising and lowering of the arms with your usual or another breathing technique. What difference do you notice?

The overall objective of yoga is the unity of body, breath and mind. Pay attention to lengthening and refining the breath when doing physical exercises. Both qualities – the long and the fine breath – have a healing effect on the body. They provide you with clarity and open up the heart to what is important.

"Open yourself up to the breath that flows within you. Receive it into your whole body. You are the breath. Observe it. Let it be and notice how the breath flows to the source. It comes and goes endlessly. That is you."

Remo Rittiner

Chapter 2. Structural yoga therapy

Guidelines and recommendations for practice

Planning and clarifying objectives

Before embarking on the selection of a yoga practice, think about what you would like to achieve. In the contents 1 of this book you will see the various core themes of the yoga programme. Select one, or more, and try it out to see whether it suits you. Ideally you will begin with the joint exercises and then proceed until you reach the neck exercises. If you have physical complaints, it makes sense to carry out the appropriate yoga practice for this regularly, over a period of four to six weeks. Plan the time of day you wish to practise. Create a yoga oasis. Do not over-extend yourself with the length of the yoga programme and your own demands. Set a realistic objective to begin with, for example, exercising 20 minutes a day or 3 times a week for 30 minutes. Early morning is an ideal time to exercise and enables you to begin the day with yoga. Find your own optimum time by trying out different times of day. Be flexible in this and be in tune with your environment. Today there are even companies that offer a special room for yoga (or gymnastics). You can of course also do yoga exercises at your place of work. Nobody will deny you this during your breaks. Even a short exercise session in between times is tolerated at some places of work.

Preparation and assistance for practising

Select a place where you will experience as little disturbance as possible. The ideal is to create a set yoga place where you will have sufficient space. Numerous types of yoga mat are on offer nowadays. Thin mats are ideal for stability, i.e. they do not slip when you are in standing postures, but they are not suitable for exercises on the knees. For kneeling exercises you should have a woollen blanket to reduce stress on the knees. You can also use this blanket to cover to keep your body warm during sitting meditation postures and the final relaxation, when your body temperature may lower. You can use a cushion or low stool for sitting in an upright position on the floor. This makes the sitting position more comfortable and optimises the alignment of the spine. However, if sitting on the floor is difficult for you, you may simply sit on a chair.

- Observe the following points when exercising:

- Should you experience severe pain, check the causes with a doctor.

- Do not exercise when you feel ill or weak. Give your body sufficient time to recovery especially after operations or procedures.

- For serious illnesses and severe mental complaints, you should only exercise under the guidance of a doctor. Find an experienced yoga therapist who will be able to give you clear instructions for practising yoga

- When pregnant it is sensible to discuss the exercises with a yoga therapist and the midwife.

- Read the first chapter, "The Foundations of Yoga Therapy" carefully before starting and integrate this into your practice.

Exercise sequences for the joints

Effects

- Promotes mobility of the joints and muscles

- Lubricates the joints and increases the circulation of the joint fluids

- Provides varied movement for the joints

- Tension and weak points in the muscles are identified and consciously changed

- Coordination of the movements of the body is harmonised

- Enables the flow of Prana life energy

- Deep-seated feelings and blockages can be released

- Prevents and eases pain from arthrosis

1. Dandasana

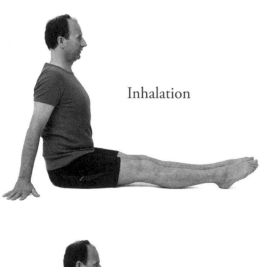

Inhalation

Effect
Bends and stretches the ankles. Extends and strengthens calves and shin muscles.

Instructions
Go into an upright sitting position with legs stretched out. Many people find it easier to keep the spine straight by sitting on a cushion.

Inhaling
Move the feet and toes forwards. This strengthens the calf muscles.

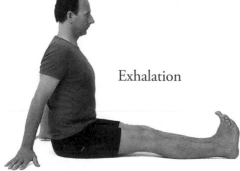

Exhalation

Exhaling
Move the feet and toes back towards your body. This strengthens the shin muscles.

Repetition: × 8-10. Then rotate the ankles a few times from left to right and from right to left.

2. Dandasana

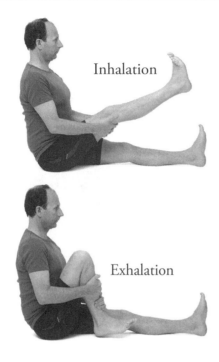

Inhalation

Exhalation

Effect
Stretches and bends the knees. Extends and strengthens the front and back of the thighs.

Instructions
Remain in an upright sitting position with legs stretched out. Hold one leg with the hands at the back of the thigh and bend it.

Inhaling
Stretch the leg forwards.

Exhaling
Bend the leg again by holding it with both hands at the back of the shin and pulling it towards the body.

Repetition: 6-8 × each leg

3. Variant of Urdhva Prasarita Padasana

Inhalation

Exhalation

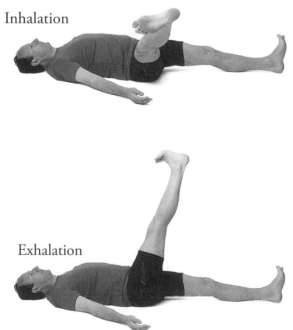

Effect
Inward and outward rotation of the hip joint. Strengthens the deep-seated buttock muscles when rotating outwards, and strengthens the outer hip muscles when rotating inwards.

Instructions
Lie on your back. The arms are stretched out next to the body. The knees are bent, the feet hip width apart and positioned close to the buttocks.

Inhaling
Lift and stretch the right leg upwards and outwards. At the same time turn the right foot outwards. Concentrate on the external rotation of the hip joint.

Exhaling
Turn the right foot slowly inwards and concentrate on the inner rotation of the hip joint when returning.

Repetition: 6-8 × each side

4. Supta Baddha Konasana

Effect
Mobilises the pelvis and the lower back. Activates the pelvic floor and stretches the groin.

Instructions
Lie on the back and bring the soles of the feet together with the legs bent. Let the knees fall outwards.

Inhaling
Hold the iliac wing (front of the hip and pelvic area) with both hands and tilt the pelvis forward. Then press the soles of the feet together and tense the pelvic floor.

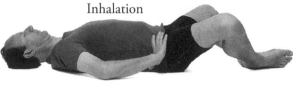

Inhalation

Exhaling
Tilt the pelvis backwards and stretch the groin area and the insides of the thighs.

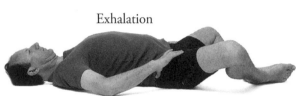

Exhalation

Repetition: × 8-10

5. Chakravakasana

Effect
Mobilises the lower, middle and upper back. Extends the erector muscles of the spine and strengthens the abdominal muscles.

Instructions
Go on to all fours. The hips and knees are aligned with one another. The hands are placed slightly in front of the shoulder joints.

Inhaling
Open the chest and raise the head a little. The neck remains long and is not clenched.

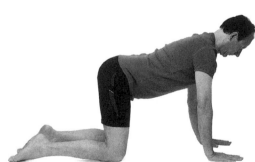

Inhalation

Exhaling
First, arch the lower back, then when breathing in, go into the starting position. Arch the middle of the back when breathing out. Inhaling, come back to the starting position. Finally, arch the upper back when breathing out.
The whole sequence × 4

Repetition: The whole sequence x 4

Note: Tense the abdominal muscles firmly to mobilise the spine.

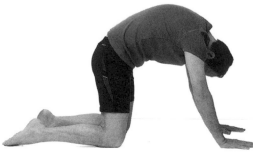

Exhalation

6. Chakravakasana

Effect
Stretches and bends the hips. Strengthens the buttock muscles and abdominals.

Instructions
Go on to all fours, hips and knees aligned. The hands are placed slightly in front of the shoulder joints.

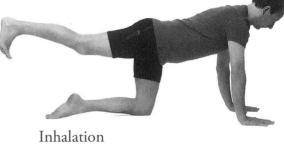

Inhalation

Inhaling
Stretch one leg backwards. Do not raise it too high (keep it horizontal) to avoid compressing the lumbar spine. The feeling of lengthening the leg and stretching the spine is more important than the height of the leg.

Exhaling
Arch the spine and bend the stretched leg. Move the knee and forehead towards the abdomen.

Repetition: 8 × each side

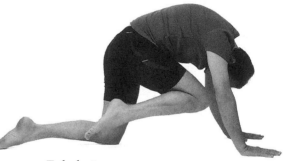

Exhalation

7. Ardha Matsyendrasana

Effect
Rotates the spine. Strengthens the deep-seated back muscles as well as mobilising the chest and ribs.

Instructions
Sit in an upright position and place the right foot inwards towards the left knee. Sit on a cushion to maintain optimum alignment of the pelvis and spine.

Inhaling
Stretch the spine and raise the left outstretched arm above your head. Support yourself with your right hand on the floor.

Exhaling
Turn your body to the right and bring the left hand on to the right knee. The right hand remains on the floor.

Repetition: 8 × each side

Note: Keep the spine as straight as possible when turning. Open up the ribs and chest. The pelvis remains stable and the twist is carried out in the thoracic spine.

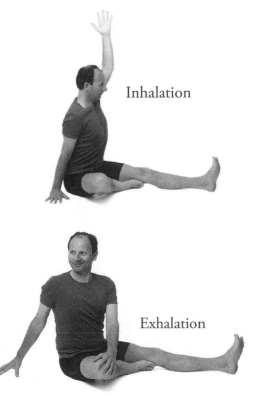

Inhalation

Exhalation

8. Dandasana

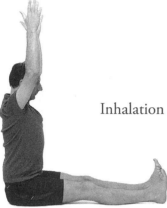

Inhalation

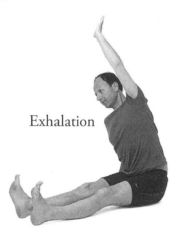

Exhalation

Effect
Strengthens the deep-seated back muscles and stretches the sides of the body.

Instructions
Remain sitting and stretch the legs outwards.

Inhaling
Stretch both arms above the head and keep the spine straight.

Exhaling
Bend slightly sideways to the right and avoid tightening up the right side of the body by not holding the position too long. Place the right hand on the floor to give support, and the left arm remains stretched up above the head.

Repetition: 8 × each side

Note: If you have back problems, bend only slightly to the side, so as not to cause discomfort.

9. Vajrasana

Inhalation

Exhalation

Effect
Stretches and bends the wrists. Mobilises the wrists.

Instructions
Go into a squat. This posture may be easier with a cushion. Stretch out the arms at shoulder height. So that the shoulders are not strained in this exercise, breathe a little less slowly and do the movements more quickly.

Inhaling
Move the fingers upwards and spread them out widely.

Exhaling
Flex the wrists and move the fingers downwards.

Repetition: × 6

10. Vajrasana

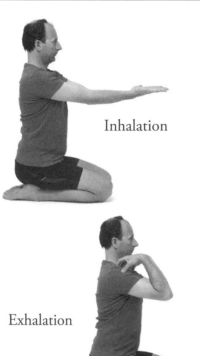

Inhalation

Exhalation

Effect
Stretches and bends the elbows. Gently strengthens the biceps.

Instructions
Go into a squat position. You may find this posture easier with a cushion. Stretch the arms forward at shoulder height.

Inhaling
Stretch the arms forward with the palms of the hands facing upwards.

Exhaling
Bend the arms and elbows and put the hands on the shoulder joints.

Repetition: × 8-10

11. Variant of Tadasana

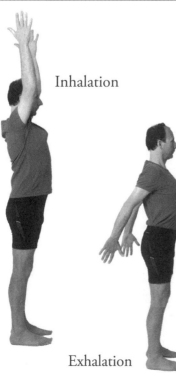

Inhalation

Exhalation

Effect
Stretches and bends the shoulder joints. Strengthens the chest muscles, upper arms and wide back muscles.

Instructions
Come into a standing position with the feet spaced hip width apart.

Inhaling
Stretch both arms forwards above the head, with the backs of the hands facing outwards.

Exhaling
Lower both arms forwards and then pull the stretched arms backwards.

Repetition: × 8-10

12. Variant of Tadasana

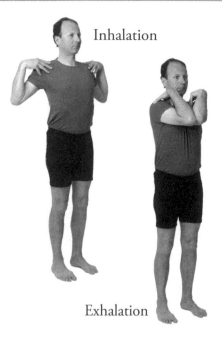

Inhalation

Exhalation

Effect
Abduction and adduction of the shoulder blades. Strengthens the delta, chest and side rib muscles.

Instructions
Place both hands on the two delta muscles in the area of the shoulder joints.

Inhaling
Move the elbows outwards and backwards. Open the chest and draw the shoulder blades in towards one another.

Exhaling
Bring the elbows together in front of the chest and draw the shoulder blades away from one another.

Repetition: × 8-10

13. Variant of Tadasana

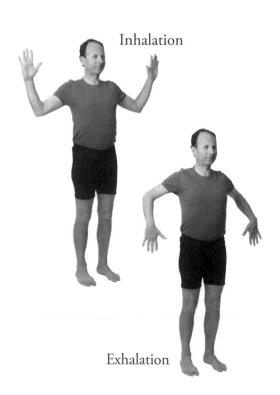

Inhalation

Exhalation

Effect
Rotates the internal and external shoulder joints. Mobilises the shoulder joints and the ribs. Strengthens the shoulder blades and chest muscles.

Instructions
Remain standing upright. The arms are next to the body.

Inhaling
Raise both arms to the sides and bend the elbows. Rotate the upper arms outwards, keeping the palms of the hands open and facing forwards. Move the shoulder blades in towards one another to open the ribcage.

Exhaling
Move the shoulder joints inwards, and the forearms and hands downwards.

Repetition: × 8-10

14. Siddhasana

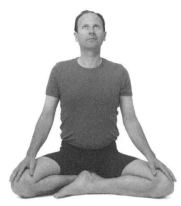

Inhalation

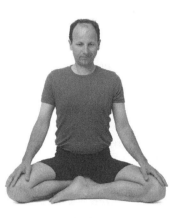

Exhalation

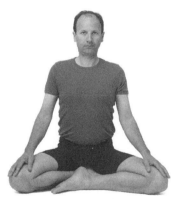

Inhalation

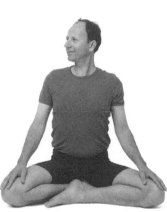

Exhalation

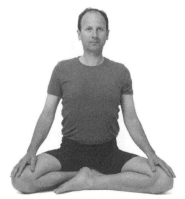

Inhalation

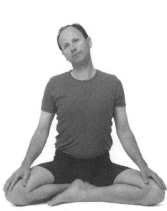

Exhalation

Effect
Mobilises, stretches and strengthens the neck.

Instructions
Come into a sitting position with crossed legs. To keep your spine as straight as possible, you may wish to sit on a cushion or chair.

Repetition: 6 × for each sequence

A. Inhaling
Raise the head and chin slightly.

Exhaling
Lower the head and chin.

B. Inhaling
Stretch the neck into a natural curve.

Exhaling
Turn the head to the right. Breathing in, move the head to the centre and on the next exhalation, turn it to the left.

Inhaling
Stretch the neck into a natural curve.

C. Exhaling
Bend the head sideways to the right. Breathing in, move the head to the centre and, exhaling, bend it sideways to the left.

Note: Do the exercises very slowly and let the breath lead the movements.

Healthy feet and steadfastness (anatomy / theory)

An architect will tell you that the structure of a building depends on a solid foundation. If the base is weak or cannot sustain the load, problems arise in the whole building. Nothing lasting can be built on a shaky bedrock.

Similarly, various pains and illnesses, such as knee and back problems or headaches can be traced back to the foundation of the body – the feet.

Our feet carry us through life. In the course of our life, it is estimated that we circumnavigate the earth around 4 to 5 times (approximately 185,000km). This marvel of anatomy, the foot, enables us as humans to walk, stand, run and jump unhindered. With its 28 bones, 31 joints, 107 ligaments and tendons and 20 of its own muscles, the foot has developed into a complex construction, which enables us to adapt to smoothly negotiating even the most uneven ground. Simply, the foot is the most heavily burdened part of the body.

Its most important multifunctional tasks include

- Cushioning the footfall

- Maintaining the balance

- Dynamic locomotion

- Balancing on uneven terrain

As with the hand, the long muscles on the foot, running down from the lower thigh, function as tendons. The muscles for this tendon are located in the lower thigh. There are also the short foot muscles. They are divided into

- The muscles in the big toe area

- The muscles in the ball of the little toe

- The muscles of the mid-foot area

- The muscles of the arch

Another very important anatomical structure is the *fascia plantaris* or tendon plate. It is the lowest layer of the feet. This tendon plate can lose its elasticity. In everyday therapeutic work, this chronic overloading often shows in the form of plantar fasciitis (inflammation of the plantar tendon) or heel spur. It is interesting that limitations in plantar mobility may often go hand in hand with shortened calf muscles (the so-called ischiocrural muscles) as well as curvature (hyperlordosis) in the lumbar and cervical spine area (frequently resistant to therapy).

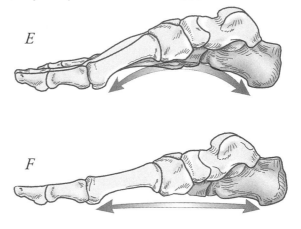

E: Healthy foot arch from medial
F: Broken foot arch from medial
Fig. 1

Various foot problems and deformities may arise due to these weaknesses in the connective tissue. Defects in the ankles from ligaments, muscles and tendons that are too weak and/or contracted, have a lasting effect on the structural form of the feet.

Inherited factors and the unfavourable effects of civilisation, such as overweight, unsuitable footwear, lack of exercise, poor ground, asphalt roads encourage these problems. Incorrect alignment of the feet can be identified from the soles of the shoes. Take a look at the condition of your soles, and particularly the differences between the left and right. *In psychosomatics there are many images for the feet*

"with both feet firmly on the ground" and "back on your feet" are just a couple of examples of this. The variety of problems includes

Skew foot, fallen arches and splay feet (these may also be combined), different toe deformities (such as hammer toes, claw feet, bunions, etc.) as well as heel spurs and pains in the tendon plate (i.e. plantar aponeurosis).

Examples

Fallen arches (*pes planus*)
Fallen arches are the forerunner to flat feet. The longitudinal arch starts to drop (with flat feet these have dropped completely). The causes are muscles and ligaments in the feet that are too weak. This results in over-extension of the ligamentous apparatus and leads to a slackness of the longitudinal arch with over-use injuries. Often, the person affected may not be able to stand using their toes. This leads to pressure marks, corns, irritations in the capsule-ligament apparatus. It may also cause damage to the knees, hips and spine and other problems.

Skew foot (*pes valgus*)
With skew foot, the mid-foot bones (inner ankle bones / ankle bones) slide inwards into the ankle area, due to weaknesses in the muscle and ligaments. The soles of the patient's shoes are often more worn on the inner side than the outer side.

Flat feet (*pes planavalgus*)
Flat feet are a combination of both the above and are often seen in practice as having developed in a similar way. This may also lead to problems in areas beyond the foot (knee, hip and spine complaints, etc).

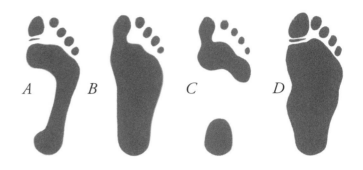

A: *Healthy foot*
B: *Flat foot*
C: *Hollow foot*
D: *Skew foot*
Fig. 2.

Halluxvalgus (bunion)
Halluxmeans big toe and *valgus*, bunion. It is usually caused by splay feet and may affect the whole statics of the forefeet. The first mid-foot bone is unstable and points inwards (medial) and the big toe pulls towards the little toe (lateral). The tip of the first mid-foot bone juts out at the inside. The foot is at its widest at that point and the shoe usually presses here. The *bursae* underneath and the skin are mechanically stressed and the result may be arthrosis.

Splay feet
The divergence of the metatarsophalangeal joints sets off a flattening or splaying of the transverse arch. The entire body weight now has to be carried on five small joints. The result is continual pain and chronic overloading. The incorrect statics of the feet and the pain of walking change the entire statics of the legs. This, in turn, leads to painful tension in the leg and back muscles.

Prerequisites for a healthy foot
Balanced muscle relationships in terms of strength and flexibility of the foot and leg muscles. In yoga, incorrect loading of the feet can be recognised in standing positions in particular. Here conscious exercising with professional help can be very useful

to begin with; as the healthy, natural foot position ultimately affects the whole axis of the legs and body. Sufficient and careful exercises, normal body weight and walking around often with bare feet, as well as appropriate footwear; these are the basic prerequisites for natural foot loading with a harmoniously trained foot that has support at four points. Happily, yoga is practised with bare feet!

The foot arch

The four-point support means the development of a harmonious, strong and flexible foot arch between the balls of the large and small toe as well as the inside and outside of the ankle, so that the entire body weight can be balanced evenly on four points when standing and moving.

Visualisation

There are four tyres underneath the balls of the large toe, small toe and the inside and outside of the an-

kle, enabling firm balancing. When walking and standing, the longitudinal and lateral arches of the foot work like a suspension system. If the connective tissue (ligaments, tendons and muscles) are weak, the arch of the foot is pressed flat and the suspension is compromised.

Setting objectives in yoga practice

- Directing perception and attention to our feet

- Mobility of the foot and toe joints

- Strong and flexible foot and leg muscles

- Healthy, strong and aligned leg-body axis

- Optimum food loading by observing the four points

Yoga programme for flat feet and fallen arches
Effects

- Awareness of optimum foot loading across three points

- Strengthens the lengthwise muscles on the arch of the foot

- Mobilises the ankles and toes

- Stretches and strengthens the leg muscles

- Stimulates circulation in the feet and legs

- Trains balance and concentration

- Grounds and centres the mind

- Deep relaxation and improved exhalation

1. Dandasana

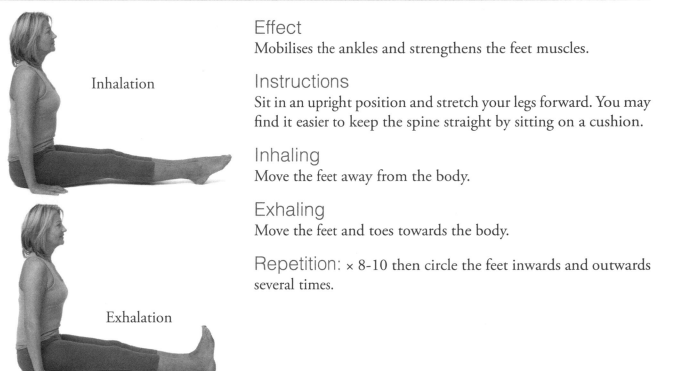

Inhalation

Exhalation

Effect
Mobilises the ankles and strengthens the feet muscles.

Instructions
Sit in an upright position and stretch your legs forward. You may find it easier to keep the spine straight by sitting on a cushion.

Inhaling
Move the feet away from the body.

Exhaling
Move the feet and toes towards the body.

Repetition: × 8-10 then circle the feet inwards and outwards several times.

2. Chakravakasana

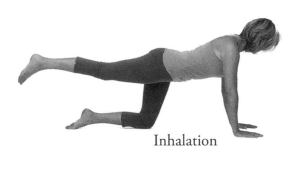

Inhalation

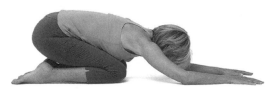

Exhalation

Effect
Strengthens and stretches the back of the leg and buttock muscles.

Instructions
Go on to all fours. The hips and knees are in alignment. The hands are placed slightly in front of the shoulder joints.

Inhaling
Raise the breastbone and stretch the right leg out behind you.

Exhaling
Place the stretched out leg back on to the floor, arch the lower back and come into a forward bend with forearms bent.

Repetition: 10 × for each leg

Note: Do not raise the outstretched leg too high, to avoid clenching the lower back.

3. Eka Pada Ustrasana

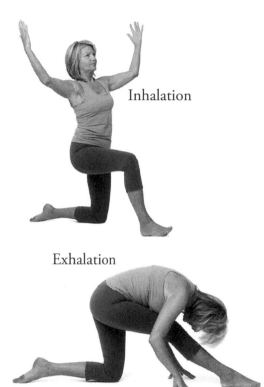

Inhalation

Exhalation

Effect
Stretches the hip flexors, backs of the legs and lower back. Strengthens the longitudinal arches of the feet and stretches the shins and the muscles at the back of the foot.

Instructions
Come into a kneeling position and place the right foot one step forward on the floor. The knee and ankle should be aligned. Place your hands on the floor.

Inhaling
Raise outstretched arms above your head and open the chest. At the same time raise all the toes of the right foot off the floor

Exhaling
Bend the upper body forwards and stretch the front leg as far as possible. Press the right heel forward and into the floor. Then place all the toes back on the floor.

Repetition: 8 × each and remain in the stretch for 3 rounds of breaths.

Note: When coming out of the posture, stretch the lower back to avoid clenching it. If you experience back pain the forward bend may be too harsh. In this case, adapt it by bending the leg forward a little and reducing the forward bend

4. Tadasana

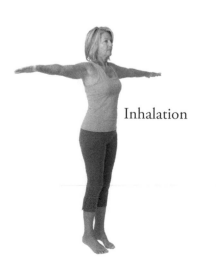

Inhalation

Effect
Optimum loading of weight on the feet, strengthens the foot muscles and encourages even weight bearing.

Instructions
Come into an upright standing position with the feet hip width apart. Be aware of the four load bearing points of the feet.

Inhaling
Raise the heels from the floor and stretch the arms out to the sides up to shoulder height. Then turn the hands so that the palms are facing upwards.

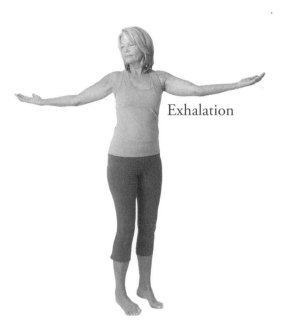

Exhalation

Exhaling
Turn the upper body and head to the right and look at the open right hand. The pelvis remains stable and rotates as little as possible.

Repetition: 6 × each

Note: Try to raise all the toes. Open the chest, leave the shoulder blades in their natural position and avoid hunching the shoulders up, which causes tension

5. Vinyasa Virabhadrasana, Parshva Uttanasana and Utthita Trikonasana

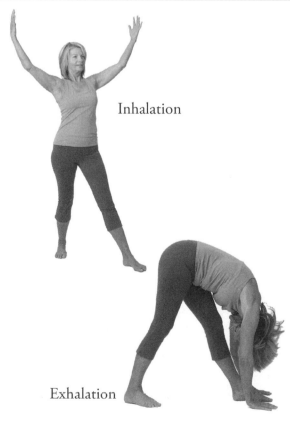

Inhalation

Exhalation

Effect
Corrects flat feet and fallen arches, strengthens the leg and hip muscles, as well as opening up the chest and sides.

Instructions
Stand upright with the legs hip width apart. Turn the right thigh outwards so that right foot points out at an angle of 45 degrees. Now take a large step forward with the left foot. Both legs are stretched.

A Inhaling
Stretch both arms up above the head. Then raise the breastbone up a little.

B Exhaling
Go into a forward bend and, if possible, place the stomach on the left thigh. Lay the hands on the floor at the side of the foot. To adapt this you can bend the left leg a little, if you have shortened leg muscles, and place the hands on the shin.

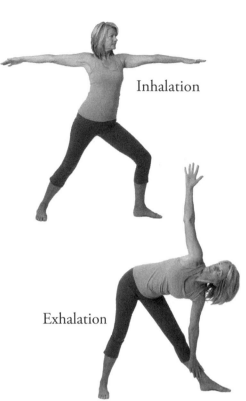

Inhalation

Exhalation

C Inhaling

Raise the upper body and stretch the arms out to the side at shoulder height. Bend the left knee and keep it aligned with the ankle.

D Exhaling

Bend the upper body forward and place the left hand on the shin. The right arm is stretched upwards. Turn the head to the right and upwards and look at the right hand. Stretch the left knee again.

Repetition: 4-6 × each side

Note: Do not do this exercise sequence if you suffer from acute back or neck pain.

6. Bhagirathasana

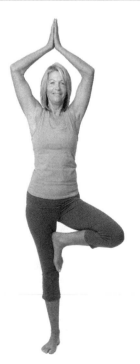

Effect

Strengthens the foot and leg muscles, and improves the balance and concentration.

Instructions

Come into an upright standing position and place the weight on the right leg.

Inhaling

Raise the left foot and place the sole of the foot on the inside of the right thigh. Move the arms out to the sides and above the head and bring the hands together over the cranium. Fixthe eyes on a point for concentration.

Repetition: Remain in the position for 6-8 breaths on each side.

Note: To adapt this you can practise the posture with the help of a wall, by supporting the buttocks and back.

7. Meditative walk

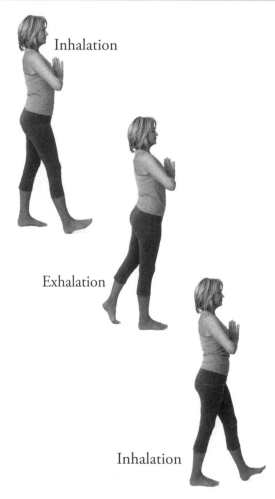

Inhalation

Exhalation

Inhalation

Effect
Releases tension from the foot muscles and mobilises the foot and toe joints. Grounds and centres the mind|.

Instructions
Stand with the feet hip width apart. Bring the palms of the hands together in front of the breastbone.

Inhaling
Take a small step forward with the right heel down and stretch the right leg.

Exhaling
Roll the right foot out and then raise the left heel from the floor.

Inhaling
Place the left heel carefully on the floor and continue in this alternating sequence.

Repetition: 2-3 minutes

Note: Proceed in slow motion and experience walking, giving the feet the greatest attention and awareness.

8. Samasthiti

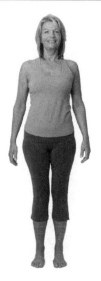

Effect
Optimum weight bearing on the feet through the four-point focus. Centres the mind and grounds you.

Instructions
Come into the standing position with both feet hip width apart. Bring the palms together in front of the breastbone. Become aware of the four points – the balls of the large and small toes and the inner and outer sides of the heel. Imagine you are standing on four tyres, each loaded equally with your weight. Inhale and exhale very consciously and be aware of the Effect on the feet.

Repetition: Remain in this posture for one minute.

9. Adho Mukha Svanasana

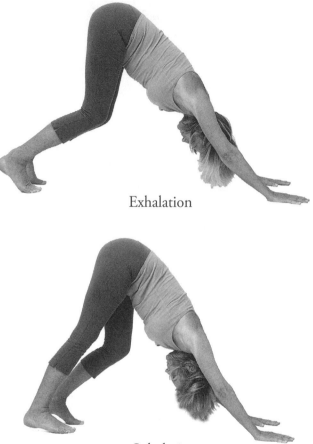

Exhalation

Inhalation

Effect
Stretches the calves, the back of the leg and the lower back.

Instructions
Come on to all fours with both hands placed slightly in front of the shoulder joints.

Exhaling
Raise the buttocks upwards, lift the knees from the floor and stretch the spine with slightly bent knees. Bend the lower back and stretch it along its length by tilting the pelvis forward.

Inhaling
Stretch the leg and bring the heel towards the floor. So as not to over-stretch the ligaments, do not bring the heel right on to the floor, even if it is possible.

Repetition: 6-8 × for each leg

Note: This exercise is too strong if you have a sensitive lower back. As an alternative, place your hands on a wall (while standing upright) and take a step back with one foot. Press the back foot into the floor and feel the stretch in the calf muscles.

10. Urdhva Prasarita Padasana

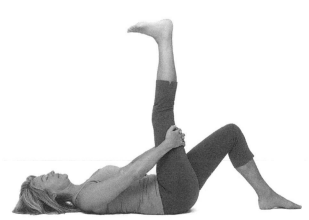

Inhalation

Effect
Energises by stretching the backs of the legs and stimulating the flow of venous blood in the legs.

Instructions
Lie on your back and place both legs hip width apart. Hold the back of the right thigh with both hands and stretch the right leg upwards.

Inhaling
Apply counter-pressure between the hands and the leg and pull it towards the body. Then stretch and energise the right leg at the same time.

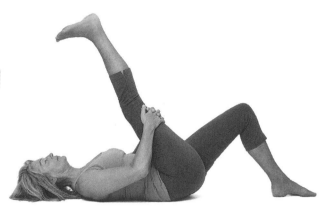

Exhalation

Exhaling
Release the pressure and pull the right leg closer to the body.

Repetition: 6 breaths for each leg

Note: To adapt this, you can bend the right knee slightly. Slight shaking of the legs is a sign of muscle tension being released.

11. Shavasana

Effect
Relaxes the body and calms the mind through lengthened exhalation.

Instructions
Lie on your back and place your hands next to your body with the palms facing up. Close your eyes. Consciously lengthen the exhalations and relaxthe leg muscles. You can let the inhalation flow freely.

Repetition: Remain in the position for 2-4 minutes.

Note: If you suffer from back pain, place your feet so that the lower back is lying flat on the floor. Or place a rolled up blanket under both knees and stretch both legs forward.

Healthy knees and stability (anatomy / theory)

The knee joint is the largest joint in our body. It is made up of three joint partners – the thigh (*condyli femoris*), the lower leg (*condyli tibialis*) and the knee-cap (*patella*). This joint is primarily a turning hinge joint which, besides bending, stretching and rolling movements on the bent knee, also enables turning movements (rotation). The unevenness (incongruence) of this relatively large joint area is balanced out by the menisci. On the one hand the knee is stabilised by the surrounding muscles, which come from the thigh and lower leg, and on the other hand by the capsule-ligament apparatus (the cruciate ligaments, the inner and outer ligaments and the surrounding articular knee capsule).

The knee has a great deal of stability in the stretched condition. However, in bent (flexed) positions it tends to be unstable.

Muscles coming from the thigh

- Front of the thigh, *sartorius* muscle (*quadriceps femoris* and *sartorius*)

- The rear muscle pulls (*ischiocrural* muscles / hamstrings)

- From the outside, the tendon plate of the tensor *fascia latae* muscle, and

- The inner thigh muscles (adductors)

Muscles coming from the lower leg

From the back of the lower leg, the two-headed calf muscles (*gastrognemius*) as well as the *plantaris* and *popliteus* muscles.

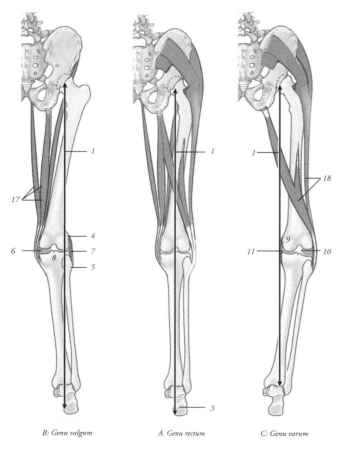

B: Genu valgum   *A. Genu rectum*   *C: Genu varum*

Fig. 3.

With a normally formed knee (*genu rectum*) a notional perpendicular runs through the middle of the head of the thigh, the middle of the knee joint and the extension through the middle of the heel bone. When there is a deviation to this perpendicular going outwards (lateral) this leads to an x shape (knock knees), and inwards to an O shape (bow legs)

Displacement

With knock knees, there is often overload on the inner tendons, outer menisci and outer joint surfaces of the thigh and lower leg. With knock knees and in a closed standing position, the insides of the knee tend to touch, while the insides of the inner ankle do not make contact. With bow legs, the outer tendons, the inner menisci and the inner cartilage-covered joint surfaces of the knee joints are stressed. When closing the legs the insides of the knees cannot be brought together. Besides this, with bow legs it is not possible to completely stretch the legs or perform the closing rotation that is so important for stable knees.

The over-stretched knee (*genu recurvatum*) can be seen frequently (in yoga in the standing positions). This may also be to do with fascial, connective tissue and muscular weaknesses or poor postural habits.

> *The following quotations from psychosomatics are well-known:*
>
> *"My knees are knocking" and "to be on your knees". The knees are the joints of my body, on which I kneel or bend but with which I can also stand up proudly. They are the gauge of my flexibility, inflexibility and humility, as well as my steadfastness to keep up my status and position."*

Pain

The most common diagnosis is knee joint arthrosis / gonarthrosis, where the cartilage layer of the knees becomes damaged. This may later lead to general inflammation, pain and reduced mobility. Damage to the menisci and ligaments is also common. This may have many causes.

The prerequisite for a pain-free and healthy knee

The good interplay of muscular chains, which enable smooth and economical movement sequences. This means that the front, inner and outer muscle chains should be harmoniously balanced (with regard to stretching and energy). What is important for a functional leg axis is the position of the feet (four-point weight bearing) as the basis for a correct knee position. Nevertheless well-aligned and mobile pelvis and hip joints are also a prerequisite for a stable knee axis. If a muscle chain is not balanced, this can disrupt the joint geometry / leg axis. Yoga therapy improves or even reinstates the functional interplay of muscular chains.

The objectives of yoga practice

- A balanced relationship between the strength and mobility of the knee, foot and hip muscles

- Strong spinal erector muscles

- Stability in the knee in different positions

- A healthy knee axis (plumb line running centrally between the hip joint, knee joint and heel-bone)

- Relaxed, flexible hip flexors

- Energetic inhalation encourages the stretching of the knee joints and the strengthening of the thigh muscles

Yoga programme for knee pain
Effects

- Corrects displacement in the knee joint

- Corrects displacement in the axis along the leg (knock knees)

- Strengthens the leg and buttock muscles

- Steadiness and stability in the knees

- Strengthens the lower back and the outer hip muscles

- Stimulates circulation

- Strengthens the back extensor muscles

- Releases tension in the hip flexors

- Improves the stability of the pelvis

- Increases the volume of breath when inhaling

1. Urdhva Prasarita Padasana

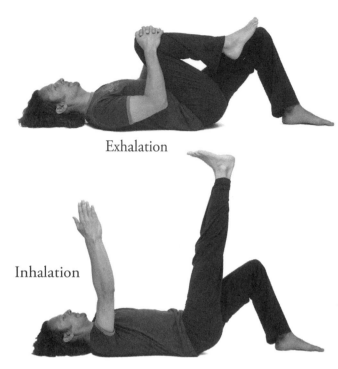

Exhalation

Inhalation

Effect
Mobilises the knee joints and stretches the leg.

Instructions
Lie on your back. The legs are bent and the feet are on the floor, tucked in close to the buttocks.

Exhaling
Pull the right knee towards the chest using both hands. If this movement hurts the knee, hold the right thigh with both hands and only carry out the movement in a range that is free of pain.

Inhaling
Raise both arms vertically and stretch the right leg upwards vertically.

Repetition: 8 × each leg

Note: To adapt this, you may bend the knee slightly if you cannot stretch out the leg fully.

2. Variant of Urdhva Prasarita Padasana

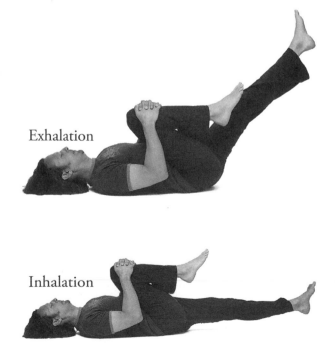

Exhalation

Inhalation

Effect
Strengthens the thigh muscles by stretching the hip flexors. Corrects pelvic misalignment by evening out muscular imbalances.

Instructions
Hold the back of the right knee using both hands and pull it towards the chest. The left leg is stretched out and the flexed foot is pointing outwards at an angle of 45°.

Exhaling
Raise the stretched out leg about 1 metre from the floor.

Inhaling
Lower the stretched out left leg slowly and hold it 5cm from the floor.

Repetition: 6-8 × for each leg

Note: If the exercise is too harsh for the lower back, do not lower the leg too far

3. Chakravakasana

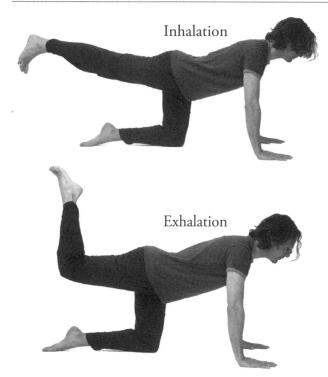

Inhalation

Exhalation

Effect
Strengthens the back of the thigh and buttock muscles.

Instructions
Come on to all fours with the hips and knees aligned. The hands are placed slightly in front of the shoulder joints.

Inhaling
Stretch the right leg backwards and flex the foot.

Exhaling
Bend the right leg and bring the heel towards the buttock.

Repetition: 8-10 × per leg

Note: Raise the leg that is stretched backwards to avoid clenching the lower back. Emphasise the length of the lower back.

4. Variant of Eka Pada Ustrasana

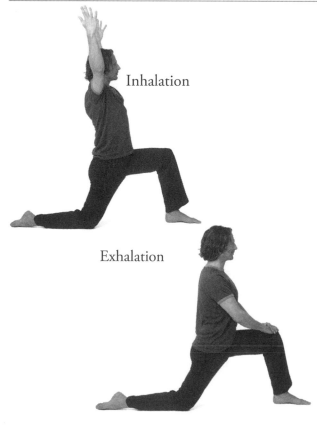

Inhalation

Exhalation

Effect
Stretch the thigh and hip flexor muscles. Stretch and strengthen the back extensor muscles.

Instructions
Come into a kneeling position and place the left foot in front of you on the floor. The knee and ankle should be aligned.

Inhaling
Raise both outstretched arms above the head and open the chest. Move the pubic bone up a little to lengthen the lower back.

Exhaling
Come forward with the upper body and place both hands on the left thigh. Then stretch the right groin. Take care that you do not curve the lower back too much by raising the pubic bone slightly.

Repetition: 8-10 × for each leg and remain in the second position for 3 breaths.

5. Tadasana and Ardha Utkatasana

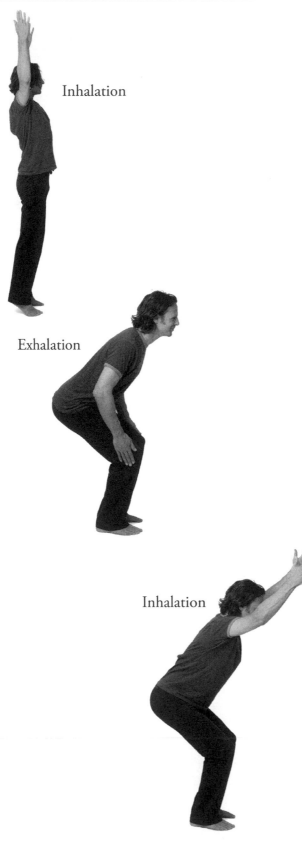

Inhalation

Exhalation

Inhalation

Effect

Corrects poor weight loading on the feet and knee joints, and strengthens the thigh and buttock muscles.

Instructions

Stand upright, feet hip width apart.

Inhaling

Raise the outstretched arms above the head and at the same time raise the heels from the floor.

Exhaling

Bend both legs and bring the buttocks backwards. Place the heels back on the floor and the hands on the outside of the thighs. Ensure that you do not move the knees too far forward (overloading). Take your weight on to the four points of the feet without skewing them inwards or outwards.

Inhaling

Stretched the arms above the head. Concentrate on energising the thighs.

Repetition: 6 × and remain in the third position for 3 breaths.

6. Prasarita Padottanasana

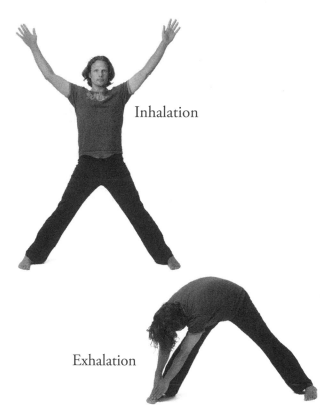

Inhalation

Exhalation

Effect
Stretches the back of the legs, the insides of the thighs and the lower back.

Instructions
Stand upright with the legs more than shoulder width apart. Set the distance of the legs so that you can feel an intense stretch in them.

Inhaling
Raise the arms out to the sides and above the head and stretch the spine.

Exhaling
Go into a forward bend with stretched back and turn the upper body to the right. Place your hands on the floor.

Repetition: 6 × each side and remain for 3 breaths each time.

Note: To adapt this, you may bend the legs slightly for the forward bend and place your hands on your shins. If you suffer from back pain, bend only slightly, supporting yourself with your hands on your thighs.

7. Variant of Utthita Eka Padangusthasana

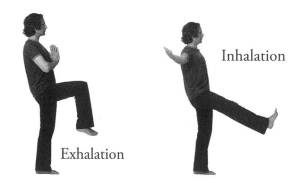

Inhalation

Exhalation

Effect
Strengthens the muscles of the feet and thighs.

Instructions
Stand upright, with the feet hip width apart.

Exhaling
Bend the right knee and raise it up to groin height. Bring the palms together in front of the breastbone.

Inhaling Stretch the right leg out as horizontally as possible and extend the arms at shoulder height.

Repetition: 8 × per leg

Note: Ensure that your spine remains erect. Should you have difficulty balancing, you may support your back against a wall. If you experience acute pain in the knees, do the exercise sitting on a chair.

8. Variant of Ardha Chandrasana

Effect
Strengthens the outer hip and leg muscles. Helps the sense of balance and stability in the pelvis.

Instructions
Come into an upright position with the legs hip width apart. Turn the right thigh 45 degrees outwards and take a step back with your right foot. Place both palms on the back of a chair.

Inhaling
Raise the right leg and at the same time raise the right arm to the side. Then turn the spine and the head to the right. Rotate the right leg inwards with the foot pointing downwards.

Exhaling
Lower the right leg and the right arm at the same time. Place the right foot on the floor. Put the right hand on the back of the chair again.

Repetition: 6 × each side and remain in the first position for 3 breaths.

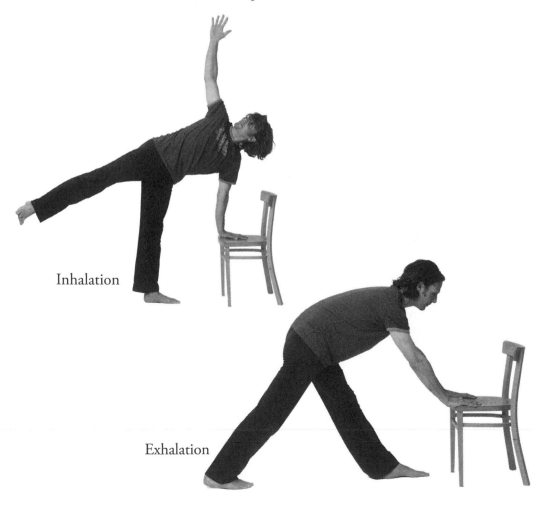

Inhalation

Exhalation

9. Shalabhasana

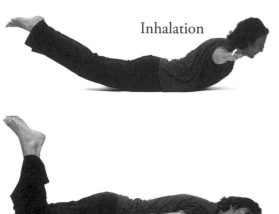

Inhalation

Exhalation

Effect
Strengthens the muscle chain, back of the thighs, buttocks and back extensor muscles.

Instructions
Lie on your front. Place the head to the right. The knees are bent and the arms are next to the body.

Inhaling
Raise the upper body from the floor and stretch the arms out to the sides. Stretch both legs back at the same time.

Exhaling
Lower the upper body, turn the head to one side and bend the legs. Place the arms next to the body again.

Repetition: × 8-10

Note: If you have back problems then lift one leg only. If this is too harsh, practise a gentle cobra pose.

10. Apanasana

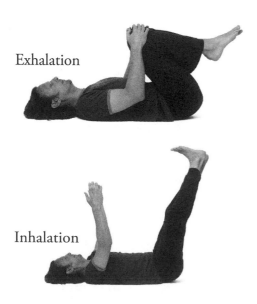

Exhalation

Inhalation

Effect
A balancing posture that relaxes and stretches the lower back.

Instructions
Lie on your back and place your feet on the floor close to your buttocks. Hold the knees with your hands.

Exhaling
Pull both knees towards your chest using your hands.

Inhaling
Stretch both arms and legs upwards vertically.

Repetition: × 8

11. Variant of Supta Prasarita Padangusthasana

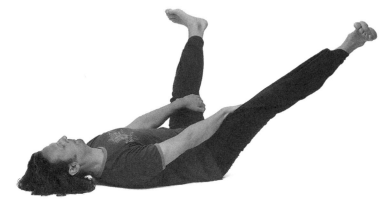

Effect
Stretches and strengthens the back and inside of the thigh muscles. Mobilises the pelvis and strengthens the pelvic floor.

Instructions
Lie on your back with the legs drawn up and the hands holding the inside of the thighs.

Inhaling
Raise the legs upwards and splay them wide. Use the hands to apply counter-pressure and tense the pelvic floor.

Exhaling
Relax the pelvic floor and release the counter-pressure. Let the legs relax and fall outwards.

Repetition: Remain for 8 breaths, then draw your legs back into the starting position.

Note: Keep the shoulder blades and sacrum on the floor, and the neck remains long. If this is difficult, place a blanket under the back of the head.

12. Shavasana

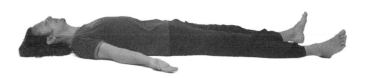

Effect
Relaxes the legs and groin area.

Instructions
Lying on your back, stretch the legs out and place the arms next to the body. Breathe consciously, concentrating on the groin area and remain in this position for 3-5 minutes.

Note: If you have back problems, place the feet up so that the back is flat on the floor, or put a rolled up blanket under the outstretched knees.

Healthy hips and freedom of movement (anatomy/theory)

The straightening up of quadrupeds into the upright position is accompanied by high static and kinetic weight-bearing requirements on the hips in terms of gravity. This also means that the muscles of the lower extremities are much more powerful than those of the upper parts. Each leg has to stabilise, hold and move a great deal of weight. It is important for the hip muscles to be in good order here (the extensors in particular) to facilitate the upright position. Good alignment of the feet, knee, hip joints and pelvis, (and of course the spine, shoulder girdle and head too) should enable a reasonable and harmonious inter-relationship in terms of the line of gravity. The hip joint allows mobility on all three axes of movement

- **Horizontal axis** flexion and extension of the legs (bending and stretching of the legs)

- **Sagittal axis** abduction and adduction of the legs (splaying and drawing in of the legs)

- **Longitudinal axis** internal and external rotation of the legs (turning of the legs inward and outward)

The hip joint (*articulatio coxae*) is a connection between the *acetabulum* and the nearby ball-shaped head of the thigh (*caput femoris*). The hip joint is encased in a very close-fitting joint capsule. The capsule-reinforced ligaments are among the strongest in the human body. The *iliofemoral* ligament, for example, has a tensile strength of approximately 350kg (the strongest ligament in the body). Part of the ligament is drawn diagonally across the joint capsule, and in such a way that it relaxes when bending (flexion) and tightens into the shape of a screw when tensing (extension). *Ligament screw action of the hip joints*

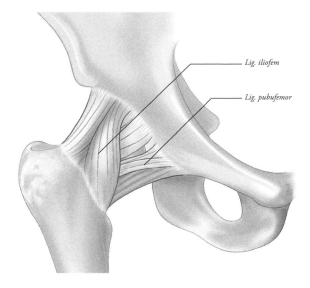

Lig. iliofem

Lig. pubufemor

Ligament tightening of the hip joint
Fig. 4.

As the hip joint has to transfer energy from the upper body to the legs, the position or angular positioning of both joint partners is important. Due to this high load, there is a growing risk of arthrosis (wear on joints) with increasing age. Greater leeway for movement is achieved through the femoral neck of the thigh bone, but this may also lead to the likelihood of fractures (particularly in old age, i.e. hip fractures). The angle of the femoral neck of the thigh bone (CCD angle) should also be mentioned here. The angle of the femoral neck in an adult is around 126 degrees. If the angle is considerably lower than 126 degrees, it is known as a *coxa vara*, and if it is greater than 126 degrees, it is known as a *coxa valga*. A *coxa valga* usually leads to bow legs (*genu varum*). A *coxa vara* tends towards knock knees (*genu valgum*) (see *Anatomy of the Knee*). This therefore shows us how significantly the position of a joint affects the resulting statics (here, knees and feet).

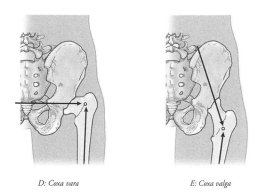

D: Coxa vara   E: Coxa valga

Balance and stability Fig. 5.

The hip joint has very powerful muscles and is a highly stable joint thanks to good osteal direction. However, being upright on two legs also brings with it considerable balance problems. Standing is principally a variable position, in which we visualise that that we do not "have" balance but must acquire it again and again. The so-called proprioceptors (sensors located in the tendons, muscles and joints) are also involved. They are part of our deep sensitivity and are important at every turn.

The most important muscles of the hips

Bending muscles (flexors) are the *ilium* (*iliacus*) muscles and the major groin muscles (*psoas major*), which together form the *iliopsoas* muscles.

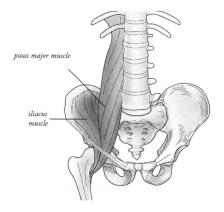

psoas major muscle

iliacus muscle

Iliopsoas muscle: consisting of iliacus muscle and psoas major muscle. Fig. 6.

Another important muscle is the *rectus femoris* muscle. It is one of the powerful *quadriceps* and can also bend in the hip joint as well as stretching in the knee joint. The *sartorius* muscle also helps with the bending of the hips. It is the longest muscle in humans.

The **stretching muscles** (extensors) also include the large buttock muscles (*gluteus maximus*, the most powerful muscles in humans), and the ischiocrural group (*bizeps femoris caput longum, semimembranosus and semitendinosus* muscles).If, for example the gluteus maximus muscles are paralysed, it is not possible to raise yourself from a squat or climb steps. The medium and small buttock muscles are the **abductors** of the legs, (*gluteus medius and minimus* muscles). At the same time they also support the inner and outer rotation of the legs. Where there is a weakness in these

Hip muscles: abductors

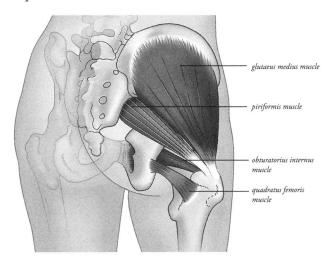

glutaeus medius muscle

piriformis muscle

obturatorius internus muscle

quadratus femoris muscle

Fig. 7

muscles, the pelvis tilts towards the side of the free leg. The result is a limping gait. The *tensor fascia latae*, with their continuous, strong, solid covering of connective tissue and the iliotibial band (*tractus iliotibiales*) ensure external stability.

Five muscles are responsible for the **adduction** of the legs following abduction, and these are known as the adductor group (*adductor longus, adductor brevis,* *adductor magnus, gracilis and pectineus).* The **inner rotators** work from the functioning of the *gluteus medius* and *minimus* as well as the *tensor fascia latae* and the *adductor magnus.* All the buttock muscles (surface and deep) that come from the pelvis and pull outward to the thigh bone (*trochanter major*), as well as all inner muscles of the thigh (all adductors except the *gracilis*) are responsible for our **rotation**.

Our pelvis, legs and hips form a unit and give us the momentum for living and locomotion. My hips therefore decide how I will proceed in life – full of energy, confidence and the flow of life or cautious, indecisive and stiff. "Maintain your composure" and "keep your balance" clearly reflect the connection of body, mind and soul.

The prerequisites for healthy hips

A balanced relationship between mobility and energy for all the muscles around the hip area. If the feet and knee statics are right, functional alignment of the hips and body is possible. Stiff hips mean more work for the back, knees and other areas of the body. If we divide the standing body into two halves, front and rear, then both should have fairly similar body volume. There should be a balanced relationship with regard to the stability and flexibility of the connective and muscle tissue.

Varied movement of the hip joints is very important. Often it is only bending and stretching that are practised, but as a ball joint the hips can do a great deal more. Rotation, abduction and adduction are just as important for the well-being of the hips as flexion and extension (three-dimensional movement).

Objectives for yoga practice

- Loosening and stretching tense and shortened hip and leg muscles

- A balanced movement radius in the hip joint in all directions and varied movement

- Powerful and flexible muscles around the hip area

- A relaxed and powerful lower back

- A balanced relationship between both iliac wings (area at the front of the hip) and a stable iliosacral joint that is sufficiently mobile

- A well-aligned leg axis from the ankle and knee to the hip joint

Yoga programme for healthy and mobile hips

Effects

- Mobilises the hip joints.

- Stretches the back, inner and outer sides of the thigh.

- Releases tension in the various hip and buttock muscles.

- Improves mobility of the iliosacral joints.

- Helps with mobility and releases tension in the lower back

1. Variant of Apanasana

Effect

Stretches and bends the hip joints. Stretches the lower back.

Instructions

Lie on your back and place the arms at the sides of the body.

Inhaling

Raise both arms and stretch them behind the head.

Exhaling

Hold the right knee with both hands and pull it towards your chest.

Repetition: 8 × each side

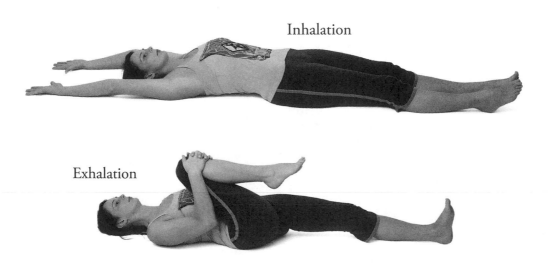

Inhalation

Exhalation

2. Variant of Urdhva Prasarita Padasana

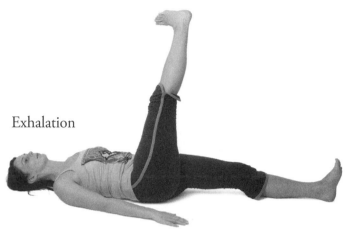

Exhalation

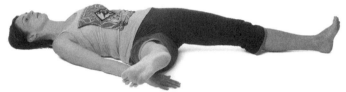

Inhalation

Effect
Increased inner and outer rotation as well as mobility of the hip joints.

Instructions
Lie on your back with the knees up and stretch the right leg upwards vertically.

Inhaling
Move the right leg outwards and point the right foot out at the same time.

Exhaling
Turn the right foot slowly inwards and move the right leg inwards.

Repetition: 8 × each side

Note: Do the outward and inward foot exercise very slowly so that the hip joint experiences as much movement as possible.

3. Vinyasa Urdhva Prasarita Padasana and Supta Prasarita Padangusthasana

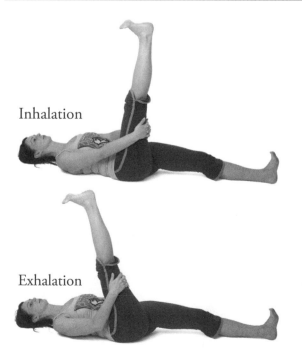

Inhalation

Exhalation

Effect
Stretches the backs of the legs and the insides and outsides of the legs (hip abductors and adductors)

Instructions
Remain lying on your back and bend the right leg. Place the right foot on the floor close to the buttock.

Inhaling
Stretch the right leg upwards. Hold it with both hands at the back of the thigh.

Exhaling
Pull the outstretched right leg towards the body. If you cannot stretch it, bend the right knee slightly.

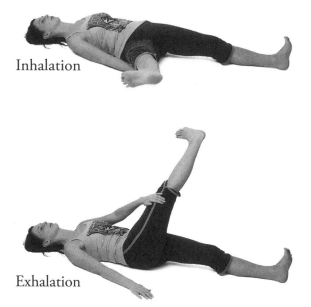

Inhalation

Exhalation

Inhaling

Guide the right outstretched leg outwards to the right. Hold the thigh with the right hand.

Exhaling

Move the right leg inwards towards the left, holding the outside of the right thigh with the left hand.

Repetition: 6 × each side

4. Eka Pada Ustrasana

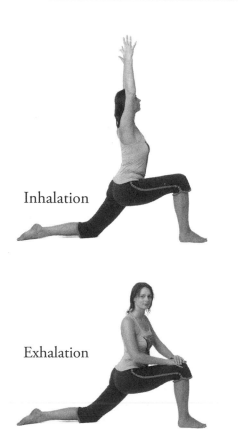

Inhalation

Exhalation

Effect

Stretches the hip flexors and thigh muscles. Extends the spine.

Instructions

Come into a kneeling position and take a step forward with the right foot. The knees and ankles should be in alignment.

Inhaling

Raise both arms above the head, stretching the spine. Extend the left groin and thigh muscles. Raise the pubic bone slightly and leave the lower back long.

Exhaling

Shift your focus to the front leg and turn the upper body to the right a little. This increases the groin extension. Place the hands on the right thigh.

Repetition: 8 × each side

Note: Avoid making too much of a hollow in the back by raising the pubic bone slightly when exhaling.

5. Adho Mukha Svanasana

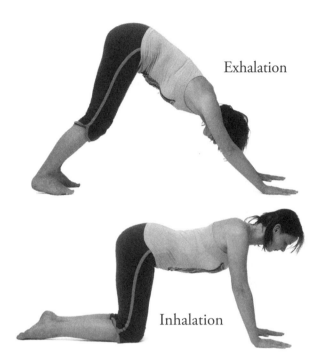

Exhalation

Inhalation

Effect
Stretches the backs of the legs and the lower back.

Instructions
Come on to all fours with both hands just in front of the shoulder joints.

Exhaling
Move the buttocks upwards and tilt the pelvis forward. Then stretch both legs. If the leg muscles are shortened you can adapt this by bending the legs slightly.

Inhaling
Come back on to all fours.

Repetition: 6 × and remain in the Dog posture for 3-4 breaths.

Note: The heels do not have to be on the floor when holding the Dog pose. It is more important to keep the length in the lower back when stretching.

6. Ardha Padma Uttanasana

Effect
Improves outer rotation in the hip joint. Stretches the inside of the thighs.

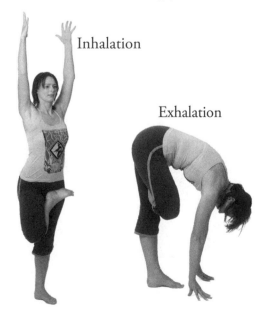

Inhalation

Exhalation

Instructions
Come into the upright standing position. Place the right foot on the left thigh.

Inhaling
Raise both arms upwards and bring the right knee outwards.

Exhaling
Move forward slowly and carefully as far as possible. The exercise should not cause any pain on the inside of the right knee. Otherwise bend the knee outwards only slightly.

Repetition: Remain in the second position for 6 breaths and go deeper into the posture in small stages.

Note: Feel whether both hips are equally mobile in the outer rotation.

7. Prasarita Padottanasana

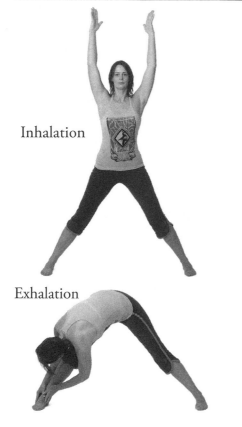

Inhalation

Exhalation

Effect
Stretches the back and the insides of the thigh muscles. Mobilises the pelvis and lower back.

Instructions
Come into a standing position and place your feet just over shoulder width apart. The feet should point 45 degrees outwards.

Inhaling
Stretch both arms outwards and upwards.

Exhaling
Bend slowly forward in the middle with a long lower back and turn the upper body towards the right leg. Place the hands next to the right foot.

Repetition: 8 × to the right and left sides

Note: If it is difficult to stretch the legs, bend the knees slightly. If you have back problems, bend forward just halfway as an intensive forward bend increases the pressure on the front discs.

8. Tadasana

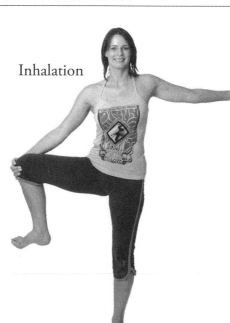

Inhalation

Effect
Stretches the abductors and adductors. Strengthens the outer hip and leg muscles.

Instructions
Come into a standing position and place the feet hip width apart.

Inhaling
Raise the bent right leg and hold the knee with the right hand. Move the right knee outward and at the same time stretch the left arm out to the left.

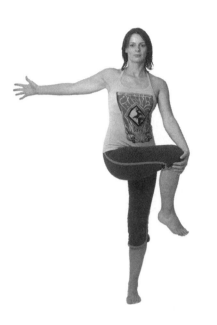

Exhaling
Move the right knee to the left and hold the right knee with the left hand. Stretch the right arm out to the right.

Repetition: 6-8 × each side and remain in the rotation for 3 breaths.

Note: The standing leg remains stretched (stable knee). Open the chest when inhaling.

9. Eka Pada Rajakapotasana

Effect
Stretches the hip flexors and deep-seated buttock muscles, which run over the sciatic nerve. Stretches the adductors.

Instructions
Kneel on the right knee and stretch the left leg out behind you. Bring the right knee out to the right. The hands remain on the floor.

Inhaling
Raise the breastbone upwards. Stretch the arms and raise the head a little.

Exhaling
Bend forwards. Place the forehead on the floor and stretch the arms forwards at the same time.

Repetition: 6 × each side, remaining in the stretch for 4 breaths

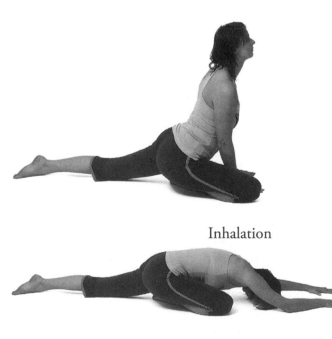

Inhalation

Exhalation

Note: This exercise may be painful if you have knee problems. In that case, bring the knee closer to the middle line and reduce the outward turn of the thigh in the hip joint. When stretching the spine during the inhalation, avoid clenching the lower back.

10. Jathara Parivritti

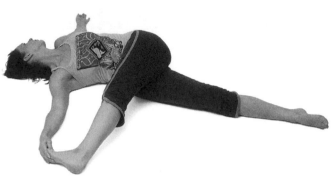

Effect
Stretches the outer hip muscles up to the knee, abdominal and rib muscles, as well as the sternocleidomastoid muscles that turn the head.

Instructions
Lie on your back with the feet on the floor close to the buttocks. Stretch the arms out to the sides with the palms facing up. Turn the knees to the right. Stretch the left leg out towards the right hand. Turn your head to the left. Pull the left foot with the right hand. Remain on each side for 6 breaths

Note: The shoulder blades remain on the floor. If you experience tension in the neck, you can place the back of the head on a blanket and reduce the turning of the head.

11. Variant of Gomukhasana

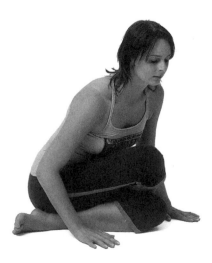

Effect
Stretches the abductors and adductors. Mobilises and moves the hips in the inner rotation.

Instructions
Come on to all fours and cross the right knee in front of the left one. Bring the feet out to the sides. Place the buttocks between the heels on the floor.

Exhaling
Bend forward carefully and remain in this position. The hands are supporting you on the floor. Remain on each side for 6 breaths

Note: You may find it easier to sit on a cushion on the floor for this pose. Take care if you have knee problems. This exercise should be avoided if you have artificial hip joints.

12. Janu Shirshasana

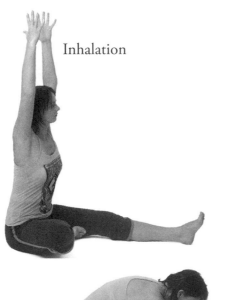

Inhalation

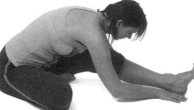

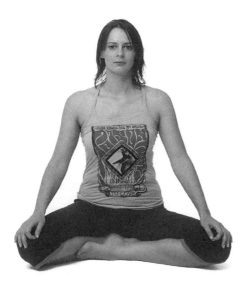

Exhalation

Effect
Stretches and balances the lower back and hips.

Instructions
Sit upright and stretch out the left leg. The right leg is bent inwards with the heel on the inside of the left thigh.

Inhaling
Stretch both arms above the head and extend the spine.

Exhaling
Bend forward with the bent left leg and place the hands on the floor.

Repetition: 6 × each side

13. Siddhasana

Effect
Relaxes the hips. Watch the breathing and the

Effect on your mind when practising this.

Instructions
Sit on a cushion. The right heel is near the cushion, the left foot is in front of the right. Straighten out the pelvis and spine. Remain in the posture for 2-3 minutes.

Note: If you find this sitting position difficult, you can sit cross-legged or on a stool.

Yoga programme for healthy and strong hips

Effects

- Improves mobility of the hip joints.

- Stability in the hips.

- Strengthens the buttock muscles and pelvic floor.

- Strengthens the front and back of the thigh.

- Stretches and strengthens the hip flexor and hip extensor muscles.

- Strengthens the lower back and abdominal muscles.

- Optimum position for the pelvis and stability for the lower back.

- Encourages steadiness and balance.

1. Variant of Urdhva Prasarita Padasana

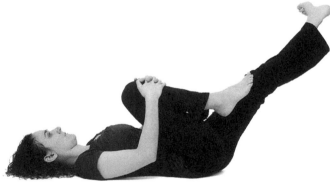

Exhalation

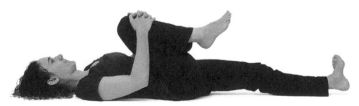

Inhalation

Effect
Strengthens by stretching the hip flexors. Strengthens the thigh muscles. Balances pelvic misalignment and differences in leg length.

Instructions
Lie on your back with the feet close to the buttocks. Hold the right knee with both hands and pull it towards the upper body. The left leg is stretched out and the left foot is turned 45 degrees outwards.

Exhaling
Raise the outstretched left leg about 1 metre from the floor.

Inhaling
Lower the left leg again to about 5cm from the floor.

Repetition: 6-8 × each side

Note: If the exercise is painful for the knees or back, you can place the outstretched leg on the floor and raise it slightly when exhaling.

2. Variant of Supta Prasarita Padangusthasana

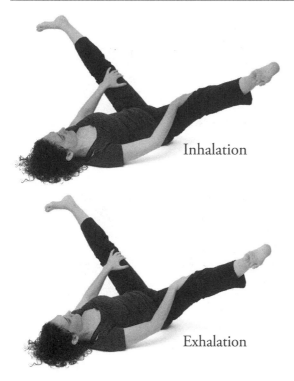

Inhalation

Exhalation

Effect
Strengthens the inside of the thighs and the pelvic floor muscles.

Instructions
Lie on your back and stretch both legs upwards. Splay the legs wide.

Inhaling
Place both hands on the inside of the thighs and apply pressure against the legs with your hands. At the same time, apply counter-pressure with the legs and tense the pelvic floor by tightening the muscles between the sitting bones.

Exhaling
Release the pressure and open your legs further outwards. Relax the pelvic floor muscles when doing this. 6-8 times

3. Variant of Chakravakasana

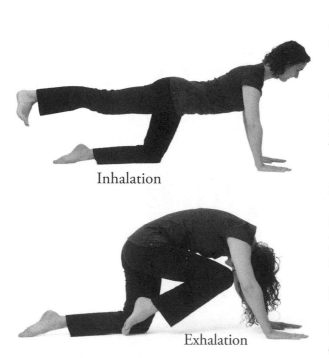

Inhalation

Exhalation

Effect
Stretches and bends the hips. Strengthens the buttock and abdominal muscles.

Instructions
Come on to all fours. The hips and knees should be in alignment. The hands are placed slightly in front of the shoulder joints.

Inhaling
Stretch the right leg backwards.

Exhaling
Round the lower back and bring the right knee towards the forehead.

Repetition: 8-10 × for each leg

Note: Do not raise the stretched leg too high, to avoid clenching the lower back.

4. Vinyasa Tadasana and Ardha Utkatasana

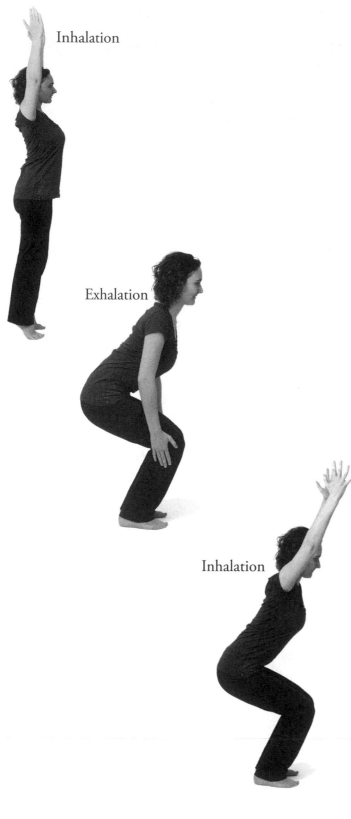

Inhalation

Exhalation

Inhalation

Effect
Strengthens the buttock, thigh and back extensor muscles.

Instructions
Come into the standing position with the feet hip width apart.

Inhaling
Stretch the arms forwards and above the head. Raise the heels from the floor at the same time.

Exhaling
Bend both legs and move the buttocks backwards. Place the heels back on the floor and place the hands at the sides of the thighs. Take care not to bring the knee too far forwards (over-straining) and place the feet with even pressure at the four points, without folding them inwards or outwards.

Inhaling
Stretch both arms above your head again. Place the weight evenly on the four points of the feet and tense the pelvic floor.

Note: Take care to keep the lower back long and avoid hollowing the back too much.

Repetition: × 6-8

5. Variant of Virabhadrasana

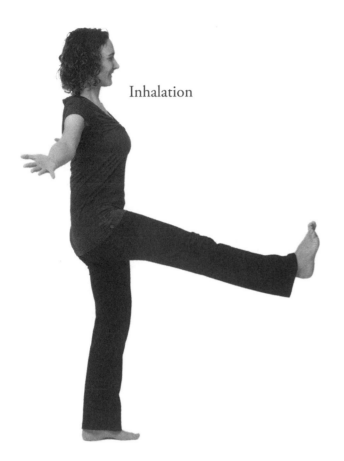

Inhalation

Effect

Strengthens the buttock and leg muscles as well as the lower back. Stabilises the hips.

Instructions

Remain in the standing position with the feet hip width apart.

Inhaling

Stretch the right leg out towards pelvis height. The left standing leg remains as stretched as possible. Stretch the arms out to the sides. Keep the spine as erect as you can.

Exhaling

Bend the upper body forwards horizontally and stretch the right leg backwards. The arms are pointing forwards.

Repetition: 6-8 × each side

Note: If you find it difficult to keep your balance, you can place one hand on the wall to support yourself. Take care to keep the pelvis stable and do not tilt too far sideways or forwards.

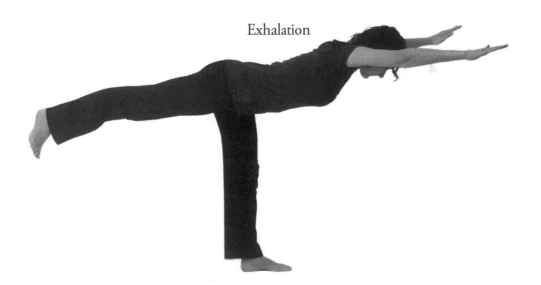

Exhalation

6. Ardha Chandrasana

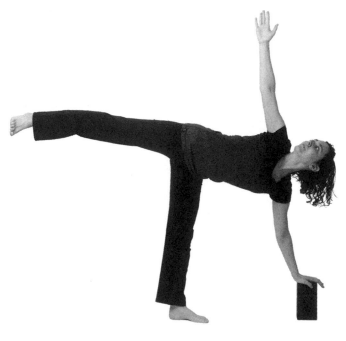

Effect
Strengthens the outer hip and leg muscles. Hip stability and balance.

Instructions
From the standing position take a big step forward with the left foot.

Exhaling
Bend forward and turn the upper body right. Then raise the right leg sideways to a horizontal position. Support your left hand using a block and stretch the right arm upwards. The head is looking towards the right hand.

Repetition: Remain for 6 breaths per leg

Note: To simplify the exercise, you can do the forward bend first when Exhaling and then raise the right leg to the side when Inhaling. If your neck is sensitive, turn the head slightly upwards

7. Uttanasana

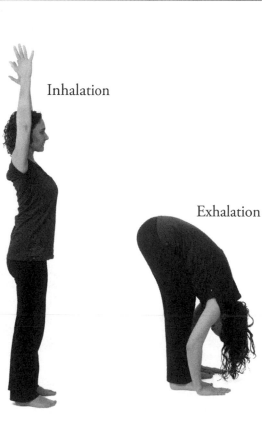

Inhalation

Exhalation

Effect
Stretches the lower back and buttock muscles.

Instructions
Remain in the standing position with the feet hip width apart.

Inhaling
Stretch the extended arms out to the sides and above the head.

Exhaling
Bend forwards with slightly bent knees and bring the arms downwards to the sides. Then place the hands on the floor.

Repetition: × 8-10

Note: If you suffer from back pain, go only halfway into the forward bend and also bend your legs. Lower the arms to the sides and place the hands on the thighs.

8. Vimanasana

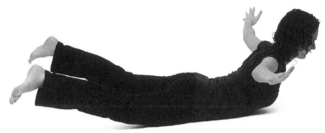

Inhalation

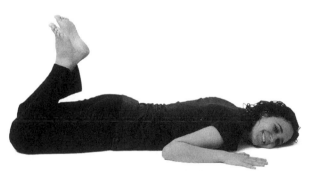

Exhalation

Effect

Strengthens the backs of the thighs and the deep-seated buttock and lower back muscles.

Instructions

Lie on your front and bend the legs. Place the hands to the sides next to the shoulders.

Inhaling

Raise the upper body and thighs from the floor. Stretch both legs wide apart. Move the arms out wide apart in front of the body. Tense the pelvic floor.

Exhaling

Bend the legs and return the upper body and thighs to the floor. Lower the arms and place the hands on the floor next to the shoulder joints.

Repetition: × 8-10

Note: If the exercise is too harsh for the lower back, do it with one leg only. With this exercise it is important to raise the body more than the legs. Should it feel uncomfortable for the lower body on the mat, you can use a folded blanket.

9. Dvipada Pitham

Inhalation

Exhalation

Effect
Strengthens the thigh, buttock and lower back muscles.

Instructions
Lie on your back. Place the feet hip width apart and close to the buttocks.

Inhaling
Raise the pelvis and spine. At the same time, bring the stretched arms upwards and out behind the head while tensing the pelvic floor.

Exhaling
Lie on your back on the floor once again, unrolling slowly. Then bring the arms back and pull the knees towards the chest using both hands.

Repetition: × 8-10

10. Navasana

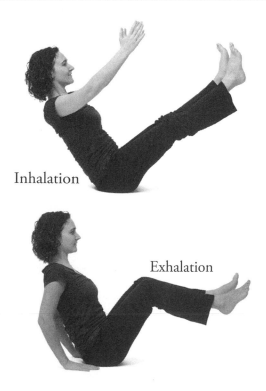

Inhalation

Exhalation

Effect
Strengthens the straight abdominals, hip flexors and thigh muscles.

Instructions
Come into an upright sitting position and place the feet close to the buttocks. Place the hands on the floor next to the buttocks.

Inhaling
Stretch both legs forwards and upwards. At the same time, stretch the arms forwards and upwards. The back remains long and stretched.

Exhaling
Bend both legs and lower the arms. Place the hands on the floor. The whole back should remain as long as possible.

Repetition: × 10-12, remaining in the first position for 3 breaths.

Note: If you experience back pain, place one foot on the floor and do the exercise with one leg only. Avoid too much rounding in the lower back by keeping the spine as stretched as possible.

11. Upavista Konasana

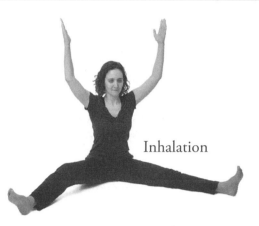

Inhalation

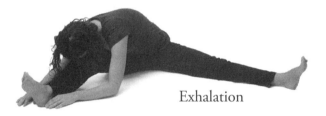

Exhalation

Effect
Stretches the lower back and pelvic floor. Stabilises the pelvis as well as the hip joints.

Instructions
Sit on the floor and splay the legs wide apart. Straighten up the pelvis and come into a natural curve.

Inhaling
Bend the right knee and raise both stretched arms to the sides and above the head.

Exhaling
Turn the upper body slightly to the right and come into a forward bend towards the right leg. If possible, rest the stomach against the right thigh and place the hands on the floor.

Repetition: 8-10 × each side

Note: If you are unable to keep an optimum alignment of the pelvis, you should sit on a cushion. Take care to stretch the lower back when bending forwards by drawing the sacrum backwards and down.

12. Siddhasana

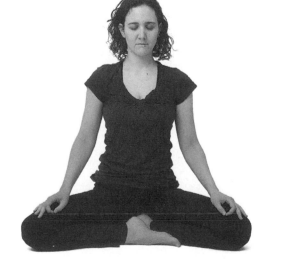

Effect
Strengthens and relaxes the pelvic floor. Stretches the hip joints, lengthens the breath and centres the mind.

Instructions
Sit on a cushion in your preferred meditation position.

Inhaling
Tense the pelvic floor and observe the feeling in the hip joints when doing this.

Exhaling
Relax the pelvic floor and observe the feeling in the hip joints. Continuously lengthen the inhalation and exhalation until you reach your limit. Note the effect on your mind after 5 to 7 minutes.

A healthy pelvis and natural posture (anatomy / theory)

"Human development from quadruped to biped meant a reorientation of the body from the horizontal to the vertical. The pelvis is the centre of the body and has a key role in the process of the body becoming erect" (1)

Our pelvis consists of the *ossa coxae* (hip bones), the *os sacrum* (sacrum) and the *os coccygis* (coccyx). The hip bones (*ossa coxae*) consist of three bones fused together, the pubic bone (*os pubis*), the ilium (*os ileum*) and the ischium (*os ischii*). From the front, the pelvic ring is enclosed by the pubic bone joint (*symphysis pubica*). From the back, the sacrum (*os sacrum*= sacred bones) connects both hip bones with its strong ligaments. From above, the weight of the erect upper body is supported evenly on the pelvis by the sacrum. The sacrum "hangs" with both its joint surfaces in the pincers of the two hip bones. The iliosacral joint (ISJ) is a joint fixed with very strong ligaments, enabling minimal room for movement. Stability, and at the same time limited flexibility, are important parameters for a healthy ISJ!

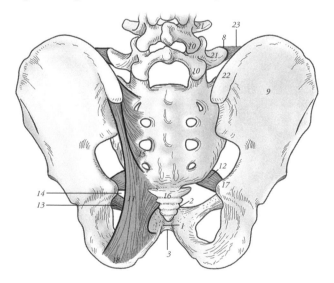

Ligaments of the pelvis from the rear.
View of the pelvis from the rear: the strong ligament apparatus is clearly visible.
Fig. 8.

Instability in the ligament apparatuses or too much tightness in the muscles often leads to blockages, in the ISJ, which are a frequent cause of lumbago. Essentially, movements and the weight of the body tend to pull on the ligaments rather than transmitting pressure to both hip bones. The result is a kind of spring system. From below, weight is evenly transmitted to the legs via both hip joints when standing or walking. When sitting, the load in the upper body rests on both sit-bones (*tuber ischiadicum*).

The spine, pelvis and legs are connected together via strong muscles. The position of the pelvis essentially affects the straightness of the spine, the balance and therefore the entire posture when walking and standing. These muscles are responsible for our being able to walk and stand upright, even when the body's centre of gravity is displaced. At the same time, mobility and stability are therefore the most important characteristics. This is why the human does not, for example, tilt to the side when walking and raising the free leg. Even in a supposedly resting, upright standing position, small impulses are constantly being sent from the pelvis to the hip joints, the lower spine, and vice versa, with signals for orientation and remaining upright. The pelvis is shaped like a funnel and serves to support the organs and innards (uterus, bladder, ovaries, intestines, etc.). Underneath, the pelvic floor muscles complete the structure and thereby support the organs of the lower body and the weight of the abdominal organs. The pelvic floor belongs to part of the muscle system that surrounds the contents of the abdomen. They work as a team as well as in opposition (synergists and antagonists) for the abdominal muscles and diaphragm.

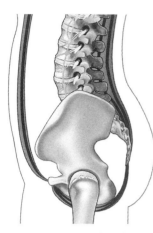

*Straight pelvis.
This is possible due to functional cooperation between the abdomen, pelvic floor and back muscles. Fig. 9.*

Important muscles that affect the position of the pelvis

a) Coming from the body
Straight, diagonal and transverse abdominal muscles, the deep-seated abdominal wall muscles (*quadratus lumborum* and *psoas major* and *minor*), from the back the long back muscles (*erector spinae*);

b) Muscles connecting the pelvis and legs
the buttock muscles (*gluteii*), the ilium muscles (*iliacus*, along with the *psoas* = the *iliopsoas*), the *rectus femoris* of the front thigh muscles as well as the abductors and adductors of the thigh and the rear *ischiocrural* muscles;

c) The pelvic floor muscles
The pelvis forms the connection between the legs and body. Due to the uprightness of the spine,

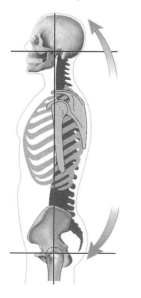

Functional spine length in the context of pelvic and cranial uprightness. Fig. 10.

humans were able to rise above animals→ became superior→ increased their capacity for survival. "Having backbone" also means possessing a footing and stability. The topics established here include the grounding and rooting of humans as well as the development of courage and strength in conflicts involving stress and threatening situations.

Preconditions for a vital pelvis and healthy iliosacral joints

A balanced ratio of strength for all the muscles surrounding the pelvis. Therefore, the muscles that come from the upper body, the muscles which pull between the pelvis and legs, the inner pelvic floor muscles and the deep buttock muscles, should be in a balanced ratio of strength and mobility with one another. This interplay between strength and flexibility enables the "centre of our body", the pelvis, to find the balance required

The objectives of yoga practice

- Awareness and consciousness of the pelvic floor

- A vital pelvic floor, i.e. relaxed and strong pelvic floor muscles

- Stable and mobile iliosacral joints

- Mobile and stable hip joints along with all surrounding hip muscles

- Strong and extended buttock muscles

- Strong trunk muscles (abdomen and lower back)

- Physiologically, optimum straightness of the pelvis and lower back

- Stable, functional and well orientated leg axes

Yoga programme for a vital pelvis and healthy iliosacral joints
Effects

- Mobilises the lower back, pelvis and iliosacral joints

- Stretches and strengthens the pelvic floor muscles

- Strengthens and stretches the deep-seated and outer buttock muscles

- Stretches the muscles in the inner and outer thigh

- Stretches and strengthens the muscles at the back of the thigh

- Improves the mobility of the hip joints in different movement directions

- Strengthens and stretches the lower back muscles

- Releases muscular and emotional tensions

1. Variant of Supta Baddha Konasana

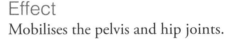

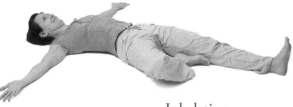

Inhalation

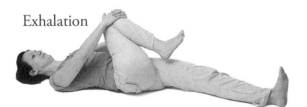

Exhalation

Effect
Mobilises the pelvis and hip joints.

Instructions
Lie on your back and place the right foot close to the buttock.

Inhaling
Stretch both arms out to the sides and place both hands on the floor, level with the shoulder joints. At the same time move the right knee outwards to the right.

Exhaling
With both hands on the outside of the right knee draw the bent right leg diagonally to the left.

Repetition: 8-10 × for each leg

2. Supta Baddha Konasana

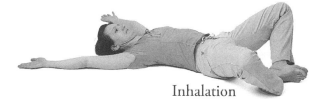

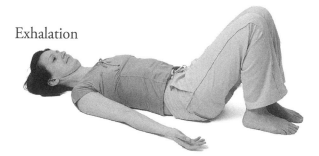

Inhalation

Exhalation

Effect
Opens up the pelvis and strengthens the pelvic floor.

Instructions
Lying on your back with the legs bent, place the soles of the feet together and move both knees outwards.

Inhaling
Slide both arms out to the sides and over the head and press the soles of the feet together. This will relax the pelvic floor.

Exhaling
Bring both arms back to the sides of the body and press the insides of the knees together. The legs are now bent again with both feet on the floor.

Repetition: × 10-12

3. Variant of Sukhasana

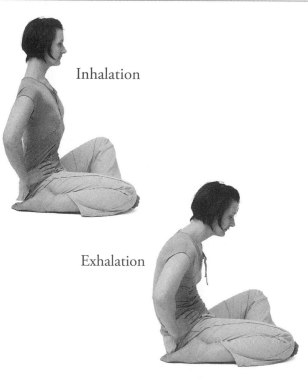

Inhalation

Exhalation

Effect
Mobilises the pelvis, hips and iliosacral joints.

Instructions
Come into a sitting position. Bend the right leg and knee backwards. The right shin and the back of the foot are stretched out to the side next to the right thigh. Place the left sole of the foot on the inside of the right thigh.

Inhaling
Hold the pelvis with both hands and tilt it forwards. Tense the pelvic floor at the same time.

Exhaling
Tilt the pelvis backwards and draw the abdominal wall inwards.

Repetition: 8-10 × each side

Note: To keep the pelvis straight, you may prefer to sit on a cushion.

4. Variant of Sukhasana

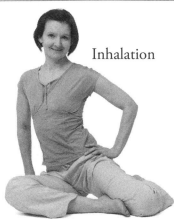

Inhalation

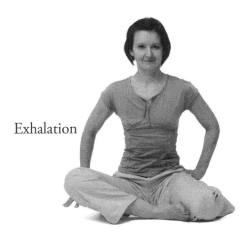

Exhalation

Effect
Inner hip rotation and strengthening of the deep-seated and outer buttock muscles.

Instructions
Come into a sitting position. Bend the left leg and knee backwards. Move the right knee outwards and place the right sole of the foot on the inside of the left thigh. Hold the left thigh bone with the left hand.

Inhaling
Turn the pelvis and left hip inwards, lengthen the spine and open the ribs.

Exhaling
Bring the pelvis and hips back into the starting position.

Repetition: 8-10 × each side

Note: To straighten the pelvis, you may wish to sit on a cushion. If you suffer from hyperlordosis (curvature of the spine), tense the pelvic floor when exhaling.

5. Ardha Uttanasana

Effect
Strengthens the buttock, back extensor muscles and leg muscles.

Instructions
Come into an upright standing position with the feet hip width apart. Bend forward when

Exhaling, with slightly bent knees and the spine stretched.

Inhaling
Stretch the arms out to the sides and come up slowly halfway with an extended spine. You can also stretch the legs.

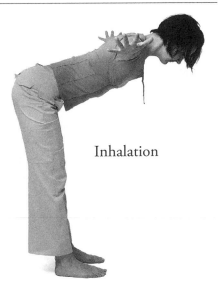

Inhalation

Exhaling

Bend forward once again with slightly bent knees and place the hands on the lower legs.

Repetition: × 8-10

Note: If the exercise is too harsh for the lower back, you can adapt it by not bending forward so far in the starting position.

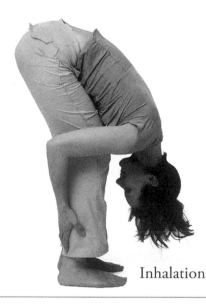

Inhalation

6. Virabhadrasana

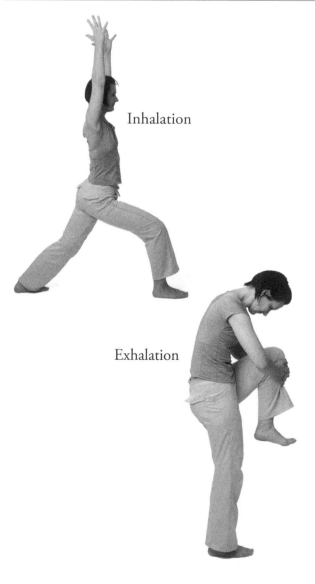

Inhalation

Exhalation

Effect

Stretches the spine and groin area as well as strengthening the outer hip, leg and abdominal muscles.

Instructions

Come into the standing position with the legs hip width apart. Turn the left leg outwards so that the foot is pointing out at an angle of 45 degrees. Now take a big step forward with the right foot and bend the right leg. The left leg is stretched.

Inhaling

Raise both arms forwards above the head and open the chest. Stretch the groin area of the rear leg and the abdominal muscles by drawing the sacrum downwards gently.

Exhaling

Raise the left leg and bring the left knee up towards the forehead. Round the upper body and hold the left knee with both hands.

Repetition: 8-10 × each side

Note: If you find it difficult to balance on one leg you can do the exercise next to a wall to support yourself.

7. Eka Pada Rajakapotasana

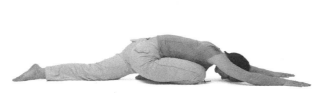

Effect
Stretches the deep-seated buttock muscles. This extends and loosens the piriformis muscle that runs above the ischial nerve.

Instructions
Come on to all fours and bring the right knee forward at shoulder width. The right heel is diagonally underneath the left groin. The right half of the buttocks is in the air.

Exhaling
Bend the upper body forwards and place the forehead on the floor. when Inhaling, tense the pelvic floor and buttock muscles and stretch the buttock muscles when Exhaling.

Repetition: Remain on each side for 6 breaths

Note: The exercise should not cause any pain in the knee joints and menisci. If you move the bent knee inwards, this decreases the strain on the knee.

8. Vimanasana

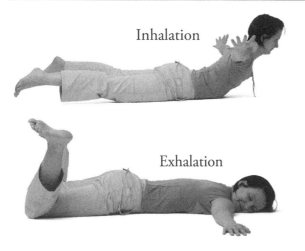

Inhalation

Exhalation

Effect
Strengthens the deep-seated buttock muscles that are important for the stability of the iliosacral joints, as well as the lower back.

Instructions
Lie on your front and place the head to the side. The arms are next to the body.

Inhaling
Lift the upper body and the splayed legs at the same time. Raise the arms to the sides up to the shoulder joints. Turn the feet outwards.

Exhaling
Lower the upper body and the bent legs to the floor at the same time. Turn the head to the side and place the arms at the sides away from the body.

Repetition: × 8-10

Note: If this exercise is too harsh for the lower back, do it on just one leg only.

9. Variant of Apanasana

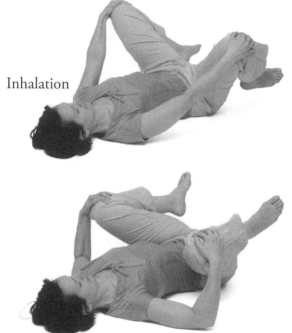

Inhalation

Exhalation

Effect
Relaxes and stretches the lower back, mobilises the pelvis and stretches the insides of the thighs.

Instructions
Lie on your back and place the feet hip width apart on the floor.

Inhaling
Hold the knees with both hands and raise the feet from the floor, whilst splaying the knees apart to open the pelvis.

Exhaling
Pull both knees towards the chest.

Repetition: × 8-10

Note: Take care that the shoulder blades stay on the floor and the neck remains long.

10. Jathara Parivritti

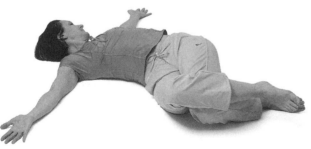

Effect
Stretches and strengthens the outer thighs, buttock and diagonal abdominal muscles.

Instructions
Lie on your back and cross the right leg over the left one. The arms are stretched out to the sides. Move both knees to the right and the head to the left when exhaling.

Inhaling
Press the legs together. Then stretch and energise the outer buttock and thigh muscles at the same time (energising through stretching). Release this counter-pressure each time when exhaling.

Repetition: Remain on each side for 6-8 breaths

Note: If you experience back pain, turn only slightly to the side. If you feel pain in the neck, turn the head only slightly to the side.

11. Upavista Konasana

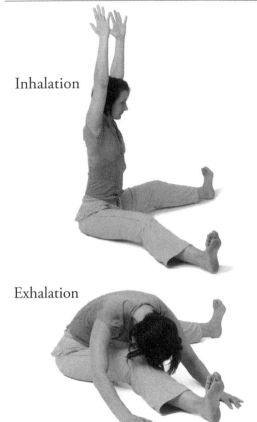

Inhalation

Exhalation

Effect

Stretches the pelvic floor and lower back. Stabilises the pelvis and hips.

Instructions

Come into a sitting position. The legs are splayed wide apart and the knees are bent. The pelvis is straight.

Inhaling

Stretch both arms forwards above the head and tense the pelvic floor.

Exhaling

Turn the upper body slightly to the right and come into a forward bend towards the right leg. If possible, place the abdomen against the right thigh and the hands to the side next to the right foot. Stretch the lower back and pelvic floor muscles.

Repetition: × 8-10

Note: If you find it difficult to keep the pelvis straight when Inhaling, sit on a cushion.

12. Shavasana

Effect
Relaxes the buttocks, sacrum and lower back.

Instructions
Lie on your back and place the feet hip width apart. Move both knees inwards so that the inside of both knees are touching.

Exhaling
Relax the lower back and the area of the iliosacral joints, which are next to the sacrum. The inhalation should remain free and the exhalation should be consciously extended.

Repetition: Remain in the posture for 3-5 minutes.

The lower back and the alignment of the spine (anatomy / theory)

The spine is the central axis of the body. It is a double S-shaped structure and is both static and dynamic in nature. Due to the erect posture of *homo sapiens*, a separation developed between the lumbar spine and the sacrum.

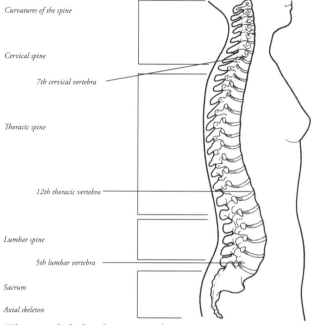

Curvatures of the spine

Cervical spine

7th cervical vertebra

Thoracic spine

12th thoracic vertebra

Lumbar spine

5th lumbar vertebra

Sacrum

Axial skeleton

The axial skeletal spine, side view (from Yoga for Wellness). Fig 11.

This lumbar-sacral area can easily be overworked and as a result, this often manifests itself as lower backache. The lumbar spine consists of 5 vertebrae and their corresponding intervertebral discs. These vertebral bodies are larger than the rest of the vertebrae because the lower section of the spinal column, along with the discs and muscles, carries the entire weight of the upper body. The upright nature of the human spine means that it must be able to carry and cushion daily loads, as well as compensating for additional asymmetric stresses or long periods of weight bearing (such as sitting for extended periods of time). Static postures in our daily lives or even repetitive movements in some sports (golf, tennis, etc.) can also create additional stresses on the spine.

One way of breaking down the structure of the lumbar spine is to think of it as consisting of two main groups of muscles, abdominal and back. However, another way of looking at it is more helpful from a therapeutic perspective and consists of what we call the local and global muscle groups.

Global musculature

The external or global system includes the vertical abdominal muscles (*rectus abdominis*), the diagonal abdominal muscles (*obliquus externus + internus*), and the long erector muscles of the back (*erector spinae*). These muscles are generally long, strong, superficial, and run between the chest and pelvis. The main function of these muscles is to regulate the movements and alignment of the spine.

Local musculature

The muscles of the internal or local system are short, located deeper in the body, and connect directly to the individual vertebral bodies. The transverse abdominal muscles (*transverse abdominis*, for example) and the sinewy muscles along the spine (such as the *multifidi*) play a particularly vital role in the local system. They enclose the vertebrae and fasten like clips to secure sections of the spine against strong shearing stresses. From a structural perspective, the local muscles are not able to influence movement or alignment of the spine. They work as a type of mini-corset (segment stabilisers) and are mainly responsible for the stability of the spine. Often, in people who suffer from pain in the lower back, the *multifidi* cannot cope with the demands of maintaining an appropriate posture. These small muscles atrophy relatively quickly, which means that they lose mass and as a result no longer have enough strength to sufficiently stabilise the lumbar spine. The effect of the leg and pelvic muscles on the lower back The pelvis is the foundation of the spinal column. More specifically, the lower back connects directly to the pelvic basin through the sacrum. The reason for the pelvic-lumbar interconnectedness is that the spine rises directly out of the sacral basin. The position of the pelvis is also affected by the muscles of the foot, lumbar spine, ilium (pelvic bone) and leg. The latter includes the inner and outer leg muscles (abductors and adductors) as well as the front and rear leg muscles (quadriceps and hamstrings). For example, both shortened hamstrings and chronically contracted abdominal muscles can lead to a flattened lumbar spine. This creates asymmetric pressure on the intervertebral discs, which can lead to compression of the anterior side of the ligaments, resulting in pain and instability.

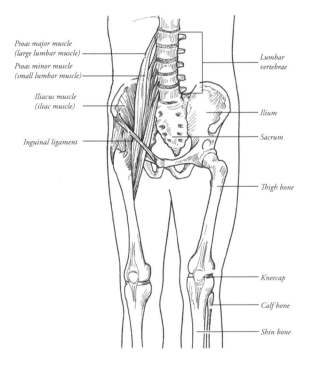

Psoas major muscle
(large lumbar muscle)

Psoas minor muscle
(small lumbar muscle)

Iliacus muscle
(iliac muscle)

Inguinal ligament

Lumbar
vertebrae

Ilium

Sacrum

Thigh bone

Kneecap

Calf bone

Shin bone

The intersection of the torso and femur via the iliopsoas (from Yoga for Wellness). Fig, 12.

Shortened muscles at the front side of the thigh / groin near the attachment to the pelvis (*iliopsoas* and *rectus femoris*) are also quite common. In today's modern world, these muscles are shortened or contracted, for many of us, due to long periods of time sitting (at desks, in cars, during meals, etc.). Unfortunately, this shortening often begins in early childhood and can lead to chronic and multifaceted problems as we get older. The *iliopsoas* is not superficially obvious so it is not very well known outside the therapeutic setting. However, it is fundamental for aligning and stabilising the spine because it provides a direct connection between the muscles of the upper body and the legs. When these muscles are shortened, the pelvis tilts forward while standing or walking. This creates an exaggerated lumbar lordosis or sway back. This imbalance in muscular tension again leads to asymmetric stresses on the vertebrae and intervertebral discs. This can lead to compression on the posterior side of the discs of the lumbar spine and resulting pain. The internal and external muscles of the thighs, buttocks, and pelvic floor have just as much biomechanical influence over the pelvic-lumbar region as the previously mentioned leg muscles. The diaphragm and the pelvic floor are also an extremely important pair of muscles for a building and sustaining a healthy back. They are functionally connected with the other muscles responsible for stabilising the lumbar spine, in such a way as to make us think of co-activation of the entire set of muscles rather than focusing on contributions from the individual muscles. Besides the complex structural system of muscles, we are also working with live, breathing people. In this approach to therapy, we cannot neglect the relationship with the breath. On the contrary, in order to truly stabilise the lower back, one must integrate the breath with the co-activation of the five muscle groups, namely the muscles of the pelvic floor, the *multifidi*, the *iliopsoas*, the transverse *abdominis*, and the diaphragm. All these components work synergistically to stabilise the spinal column. The concept of natural lordosis or curvature is often confused with a hyper-lordosis or sway back. Natural lordosis is essential for avoiding back problems in our daily life. This is only possible when we are able to sustain a structurally balanced system. However, in modern times, imbalance is more often the norm in daily life. These problems result in poor posture and muscular imbalance for many people (i.e. sway back, tight lower back, or acquired scoliosis). Again, these can lead to structural wear and tear, such as a limited range of motion for the small vertebral joints, ruptured or bulging discs, slipped discs, irritation of the nerves.

"The spine is the physical and spiritual support structure. It upholds and protects me in all situations in life. Without it, I would break down." Problems in the lumbar spine area often reflect mental conflicts such as worry and uncertainty, irrespective of whether these are material or emotional. In the vernacular, the back and its rigidity are used to symbolise more than a bony structure in the body

"To back someone up; to stab someone in the back; to be unbending (or unyielding); to have your back against the wall."

Prerequisites for a healthy lower back

The architecture of the human body should be seen as that of a stable building, i.e. how it is built from top to bottom (the foundation / the feet / the legs / the pelvis / the spine / the shoulder girdle / the cervical spine / the head). So, for example, problems in the lower back can sometimes be traced back to structural issues in the feet, knees or pelvis. Due to the interconnectedness of muscles used to perform complex movements, the pain manifested from one physical problem may be felt at a completely different location in the body, for example the lower back.

Objectives

Yoga therapy is concerned with establishing flexibility and stability in the muscles, in order to create space in the passive structures (spine, intervertebral discs, nerves, etc.). Reprogramming unconscious breathing habits into a more conscious and relaxed breath, also known as breath awareness, is fundamental for developing fluid and relaxed movement.

- Extending and lengthening the lumbar spine
- Stretching the hip flexors
- Lengthening and relaxing the abdominal and back muscles
- A harmonious interaction between strength and flexibility in the muscles of the legs, pelvis and trunk
- Conscious and harmonious breathing
- Learning from healthy movements and postures

Yoga programme for a relaxed lower back

Effects

- Stretches the hip flexors and groin muscles.

- Strengthens and relaxes the muscles of the pelvic floor.

- Stretches and relaxes the abdominal muscles.

- Mobilises and stretches the lower back.

- Strengthens the buttocks and back extensor muscles

- Stretches and straightens the spine.

- Stretches the insides and back of the legs.

- Strengthens the leg and abdominal muscles.

- Stretches the outer hip and deep-seated buttock muscles.

- Awareness of natural lordosis (curvature) and healthy movement in the lower back.

- Extended exhalation and deep relaxation

1. Variant of Shavasana

Inhalation

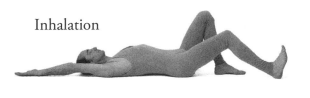

Exhalation

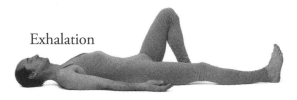

Effect
Stretches the spine and strengthens the pelvic floor. Relaxes the lower back muscles.

Instructions
Lie on your back with the right leg stretched out and the left leg bent with the foot on the floor. Place the arms to the sides next to the body. The palms are facing upwards.

Inhaling
Press the right heel to the floor and tense the pelvic floor. Bend the right knee slightly and stretch the right arm above the head.

Exhaling
Take the right arm backwards and let the lower back rest into the floor. Stretch the right leg again.

Repetition: 8 × each side

2. Supta Baddha Konasana

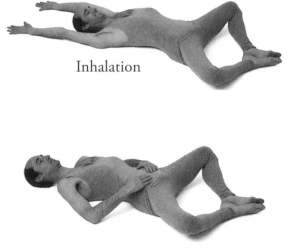

Inhalation

Exhalation

Effect

Stretches the groin area. Strengthens the pelvic floor and the deep buttock muscles.

Instructions

Lying on your back, bring the soles of the feet together and move the knees outwards.

Inhaling

Press the soles of the feet together to activate the pelvic floor. At the same time, stretch both arms above the head.

Exhaling

Bring both hands on to the groin and relax the pelvic floor. Open the knees further outwards.

Repetition: 8-10 times

Note: If you feel pain in the lower back during this exercise, move the knees only slightly outwards.

3. Variant of Jathara Parivritti

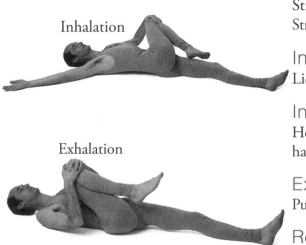

Inhalation

Exhalation

Effect

Stretches the outer hip and the deep-seated buttock muscles. Stretches the diagonal abdominal muscles and the side rib muscles.

Instructions

Lie on your back and place the right foot close to the buttock.

Inhaling

Hold the right knee outward and pull it to the left using the left hand. Stretch the right arm upwards along the floor.

Exhaling

Pull the right knee towards the right of the chest using both hands.

Repetition: 8 × each side

4. Eka Pada Ustrasana

Effect
Stretches the hip flexors and abdominal muscles. Strengthens the deep-seated back extensor muscles and the spine. Mobilises the thoracic spine.

Instructions
Come on to your knees. Step the right foot forward so that the shin is vertical.

Inhaling
Lift both arms in a V above the head and stretch the spine. Raise the breastbone and open the chest.

Exhaling
Turn the upper body to the right and bring the left hand to the right knee and the right hand to the sacrum.

Repetition: 8 × each side

Note: When stretching ensure a natural curvature but avoid over-bending in the lower back. Make sure you do not tilt the pelvis forward during the stretch. Activate the abdominal muscles and keep the pelvis straight. Feel a stretch in the left hip flexors and thigh muscles.

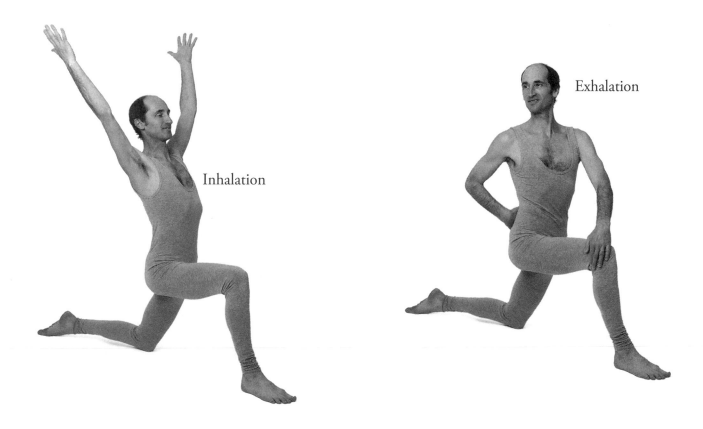

Inhalation

Exhalation

5. Variant of Chakravakasana

Effect
Stretches the spine and strengthens the muscle chain:
back of the thigh, buttocks and back muscles. Mobilises the spine and strengthens the straight abdominal muscles.

Instructions
Come on to all fours. The hips and knees are in alignment. The hands are placed slightly in front of the shoulder joints.

Inhaling
Stretch the right leg out horizontally to the rear.

Exhaling
Round the lower back and bring the right knee towards the forehead, so that you are activating the abdominal muscles.

Repetition: 8-10 × for each leg

Note: Do not raise the leg too high, to avoid clenching in the lower back area. Pay more attention to stretching the lower back.

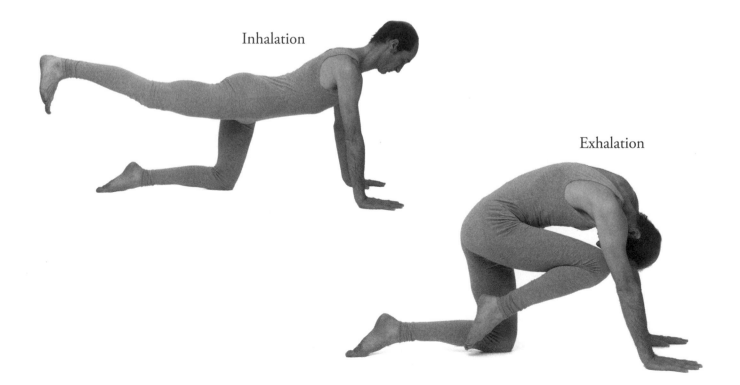

Inhalation

Exhalation

6. Vinyasa Tadasana and Ardha Uttananasa

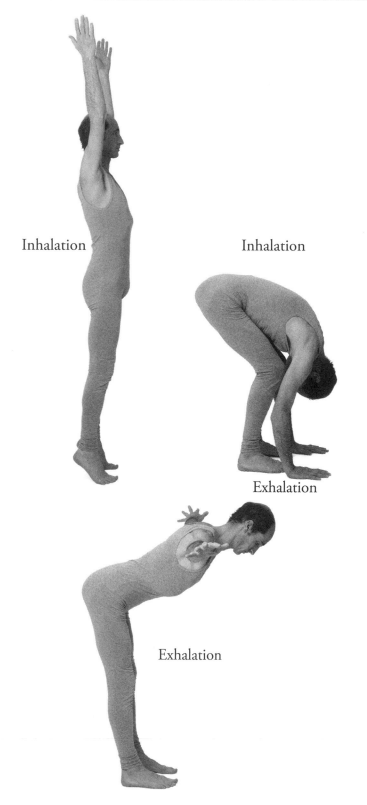

Inhalation

Inhalation

Exhalation

Exhalation

Effect
Stretches and strengthens the lower back.

Instructions
Come into the upright standing position with the feet hip width apart.

Inhaling
Raise the heels from the floor and stretch the arms in front of the body above the head.

Exhaling
Lower the heels and come into the forward bend with bent knees. Place the stomach on the thighs and the hands, if possible, on the floor.

Inhaling
Raise the head slightly, stretch the spine and raise the upper body half way up with arms to the sides. Stretch the legs if possible. Then return to the second position when exhaling.

and back to the starting position inhaling.

Repetition: 6 × and remain in the second position for 3 breaths at the end.

Note: If you experience back pain, bend forward only slightly and place the hands on the thighs. The third position can simply be left out.

7. Virabhadrasana and Ardha Parshva Uttanasana

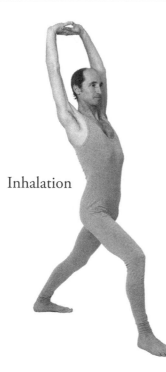

Inhalation

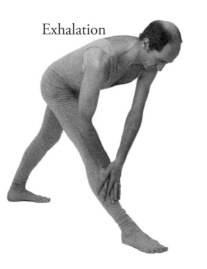

Exhalation

Effect

Stretches the upper hip flexors and strengthens the back extensor muscles. Extends the lower back and the backs of the thighs. Strengthens the thigh muscles.

Instructions

In the upright standing position, turn the left leg outwards, so that the left foot is pointing out at 45 degrees. Now take a big step forward with the right foot. Align both hips forwards and bend the right leg.

Inhaling

Interlace the fingers and stretch the arms upwards above the head. The palms are facing upwards.

Exhaling

Come into the half forward bend with a stretched spine and place the hands on the shin of the front stretched leg.

Repetition: 8 × each side

Note: If the forward bend is painful, only take the movement up to the point where there is no pain.

8. Prasarita Padottanasana

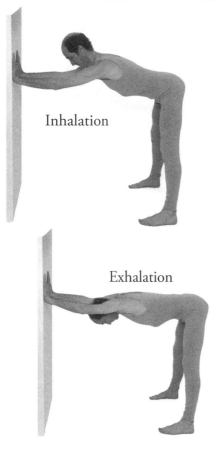

Inhalation

Exhalation

Effect
Stretches the muscles on the insides of the thighs and lower back. Stretches the spine and strengthens the lower back.

Instructions
Stand in front of a wall and push against the wall with the hands. Position the feet wide apart in a straddling position. Then come into the half forward bend.

Inhaling
Raise the head and upper body with the spine extended. Open the chest. The hands remain against the wall.

Exhaling
Lower the upper body with the spine stretched into a horizontal position and stretch the back and insides of the thighs.

Repetition: 8-10 times, remaining in the second position for 3 breaths

9. Chakravakasana

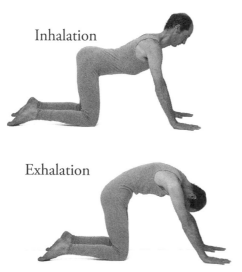

Inhalation

Exhalation

Effect
One-sided stretching and mobilisation of the lower back. Releases tension in the lower back and buttocks.

Instructions
Come on to all fours, with hips and knees aligned. Place the right knee about 10 cm in front of the left knee. The hands are placed slightly in front of the shoulder joints.

Inhaling
Open the chest. The neck remains long and the lower back is in a natural curvature.

Exhaling
Round the lower back and stretch it. Activate the abdominal muscles and pull the navel in towards the spine.

Repetition: 8-10 × each side

10. Dvipada Pitham and Apanasana

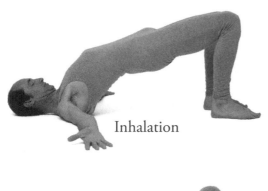

Inhalation

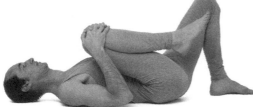

Exhalation

Effect
Strengthens and stretches the back and buttocks.

Instructions
Lie on your back and place the feet hip width apart close to the buttocks.

Inhaling
Raise the pelvis and bring the arms to the sides at the same time. Open the chest.

Exhaling
Place the back and buttocks on the floor again and use both hands to draw the right knee towards the chest.

Repetition: 8-10 × each side

11. Apanasana

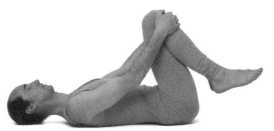

Inhalation

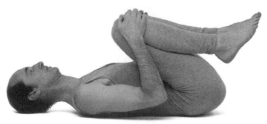

Exhalation

Effect
Stretches the lower back and buttocks. Deeper, longer exhalation and relaxing of the nervous system with deep sounds.

Instructions
Lying on your back, pull your feet up and hold the knees with both hands.

Inhaling
Stretch the arms and the knees away from the chest.

Exhaling
Pull the knees slowly back to the chest. At the same time make a deep "ooh" sound

Repetition: × 10

12. Shavasana

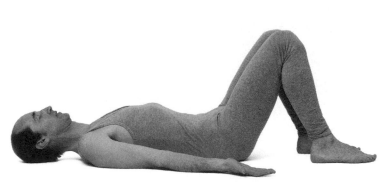

Effect
Relaxes the lower back and abdominal area. Deepened breathing and relaxation of the nervous system. Mindfulness through watching the breath.

Instructions
Lie on your back and place the arms next to the body. Take a minute to become aware of the lower back. Then observe the movement of the abdominal wall for 3-5 minutes.

Note: If the back is hurting, place the feet close to the buttocks, so that the lower back is flat on the floor. If it is more comfortable for the lower back, place a rolled up blanket under the knees and stretch the legs forwards.

Yoga practice for a strong lower back
Objectives

- Increases mobility in the lower back

- Stabilises the muscles of lower back and supports the natural alignment of the spine

- Stretches the muscles of the thighs and hip flexors

- Strengthens the buttocks and deep-seated back muscles

- Strengthens the pelvic floor

- Increases the breathing capacity and supply of oxygen

- Energises and strengthens the body, breath and mind

1. Urdhva Prasarita Padasana

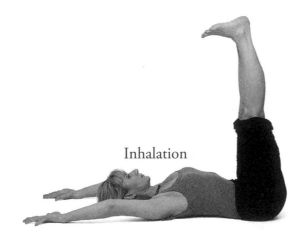

Inhalation

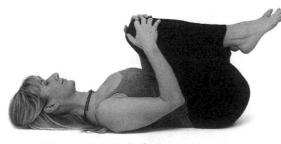

Exhalation

Effect
Lengthens and stretches the back and hamstrings

Instructions
Lie on your back and lift the legs, knees bent, off of the floor. Let the arms rest on the floor next to your body, with the palms towards the floor.

Inhaling
Lift both arms straight up and bring them on to the floor behind your head. At the same time bring both legs up vertically. Stretch the spine by extending through your arms and legs.

Exhaling
Use the hands to pull both knees towards the chest.

Repetition: × 8-10

2. Urdhva Prasarita Padasana

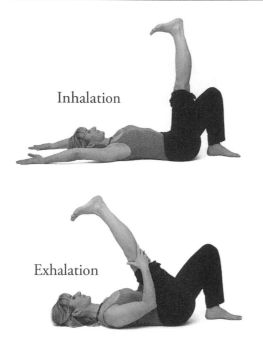

Inhalation

Exhalation

Effect
Stretches the back of the legs and the lower back.

Instructions
Lie on your back and bring the feet flat on to the floor with the knees bent. Place the arms by your sides on the floor.

Inhaling
Lift both arms up and then on to the floor behind your head, and at the same time, straighten the right leg upwards.

Exhaling
Bring the hands to the back of the right thigh and gently pull the straightened leg towards the body.

Repetition: 8 × each side

3. Eka Pada Ustrasana

Effect
Stretches the front of the thigh and the hip flexors. Opens the chest and ribs.

Instructions
Kneel and place your right foot on the floor in front of you. The knee is directly above the ankle. Bend the left knee and reach the hands behind you, holding on somewhere above the left ankle. Gently pull the left foot toward the buttocks.

Inhaling
Activate the muscles of the pelvic floor and the right thigh. Let the breath stretch the chest.

Exhaling
Bring the groin slightly forward without creating an excessive lumbar curve. Stretch the left thigh.

Repetition
Remain on each side for 6 breaths

Note:
Exhaling, lift the public bone slightly to stretch the groin effectively. This also helps to stabilise and protect the lower back. If kneeling causes pain in the knee cap, you can place a blanket under the rear knee. If this is not sufficient, then place the shin of the rear leg on to the floor and let the arms hang next to the body.

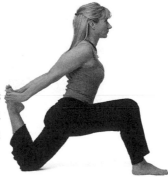

4. Vinyasa Tadasana und Ardha Utkatasana

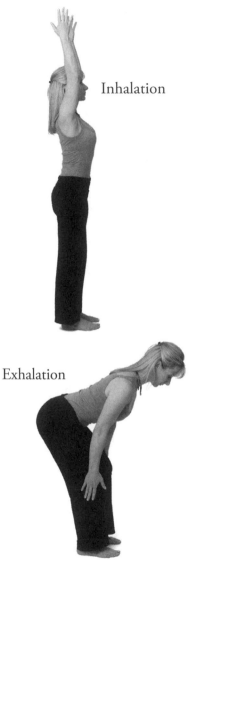

Inhalation

Exhalation

Effect
Strengthen the buttocks, thighs and erector muscles of the back

Instructions
Come into the standing position with the feet hip width apart.

Inhaling
Lift the straight arms forward and up above the head.

Exhaling
Bend both knees and let the buttocks sink. Bring your hands to the outside of the thighs. Make sure the knees stay above the ankles.

Inhaling
Lift both straight arms over the head while keeping the lower part of the body in the same position. Pay attention to ensuring the knees are above the ankles and distribute the weight evenly across the feet. Engage the muscles of the pelvic floor.

Repetition: 6 × and stay in the second position for 3 breaths. Remain in the final position for 3 breaths.

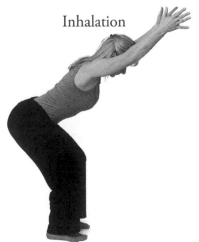

Inhalation

5. Variant of Virabhadrasana

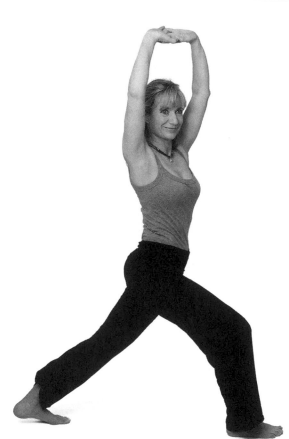

Effect
Strengthens the erector muscles of the spine. Strengthens by extending the transverse abdominal muscle and hip flexors.

Instructions
In the standing position, turn the left foot 45 degrees outwards. Lift the heel slightly off the floor. Step the right foot forward with a big step and bend the right leg.

Inhaling, raise both arms above the head, interlacing the fingers with the palms turned upwards. Use the extension in the arms to help create axial extension in the spine and stretch the front of the body.

Exhaling
Turn the upper body and the spine slightly to the right. Stretch the left hip flexor and transverse abdominal muscles.

Repetition: Remain on each side for 6 breaths.

Note: Pay careful attention to the natural curve of the lower back and the optimum extension of the spine.

6. Vinyasa Virabhadrasana and Parshva Uttanasana

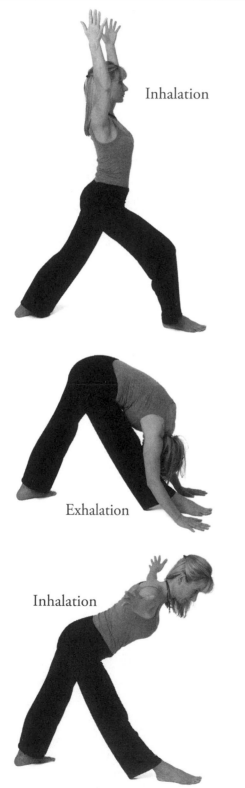

Inhalation

Exhalation

Inhalation

Effect
Stretches and strengthens the lower back and buttocks. Mobilises and stabilises the lower back.

Instructions
Use the same starting posture as in the last exercise. This time, step the right foot about 6 inches further forward and let the left heel touch the floor.

Inhaling
Bring the straight arms out to the side and over the head with the palms of your hands facing one another.

Exhaling
Bend forward, straighten the right leg and fold the body forward. If possible, bring the hands to the floor on either side of the right foot. If the hands cannot easily come to the ground with the front leg straight, bend the front leg until you are comfortably touching the ground.

Inhaling
First, raise your chest and head to extend the spine. Then, lift your upper body half way up to the standing position, with your arms out wide to the sides, at the same height as your shoulders.

Repetition: 6 × each side

Note: To avoid potential back strain, only go as far into the forward bend as is comfortable for your body.

7. Uttanasana

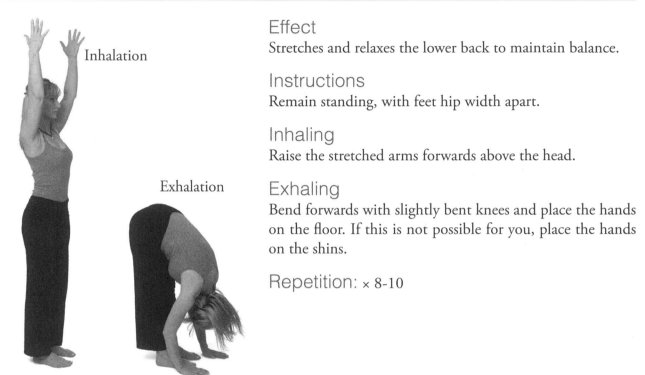

Inhalation

Exhalation

Effect
Stretches and relaxes the lower back to maintain balance.

Instructions
Remain standing, with feet hip width apart.

Inhaling
Raise the stretched arms forwards above the head.

Exhaling
Bend forwards with slightly bent knees and place the hands on the floor. If this is not possible for you, place the hands on the shins.

Repetition: × 8-10

8. Bhujangasana

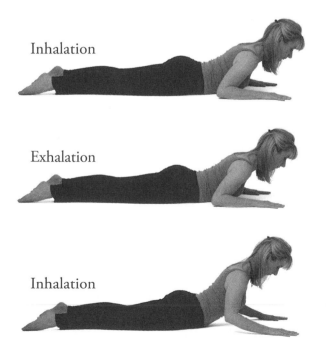

Inhalation

Exhalation

Inhalation

Effect
Strengthens the deep-seated back extensor muscles.

Instructions
Lie on your stomach with the hands next to the shoulder joints. The head is on the floor turned to one side.

Inhaling
Using the strength of the back, raise the head and chest slightly. In doing this there should be little pressure on the hands.

Exhaling
Remain in the holding position.

Inhaling
Go a little higher.

Repetition: Remain in the third position for 4-6 breaths.

Note: Do not press yourself higher using the hands. Find a natural curvature and lengthen the spine. Respect your limits and watch the breath.

9. Ardha Shalabhasana / Vimanasana

Inhalation

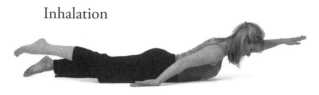

Exhalation

Inhalation

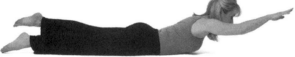

Exhalation

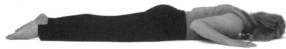

Inhalation

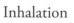
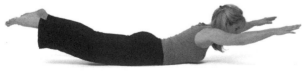

Exhalation

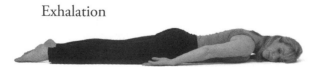

Effect
Strengthens the back and the deep buttock muscles.

Instructions
Remain lying on your stomach. Place the arms next to the body. The head is on the floor and turned to one side.

Inhaling
Raise the head, chest, right leg and left arm at the same time.

Exhaling
Lower the chest and place the left arm next to the body. Turn the head to the right.

Inhaling
Raise the head, chest, left leg and right arm at the same time.

Exhaling
Lower the chest and place the right arm next to the body. Turn the head to the left.

Inhaling
Raise the head, chest, and both legs at the same time. The legs are splayed apart. Stretch the arms forward and leave the shoulders relaxed.

Exhaling
Lower the upper body and legs. Move the arms to the sides of the body, turn the head to the right and rest it down.

Repetition: 6 × for the entire sequence

10. Apanasana

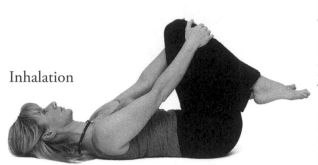

Inhalation

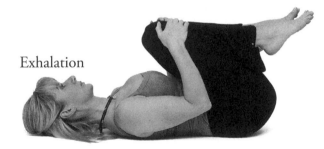

Exhalation

Effect
Stretches the lower back and loosens the neck muscles.

Instructions
Lie on your back with the feet flat on the floor and knees up. The feet are hip width apart.

Inhaling
Raise the feet from the floor and hold the knees with both hands. The arms are stretched.

Exhaling
Pull both knees towards the chest.

Repetition: × 10

Note: Keep the shoulder blades on the floor and move the knees forwards Inhaling. If this clenches your neck, place a folded blanket under the back of the head.

11. Navasana

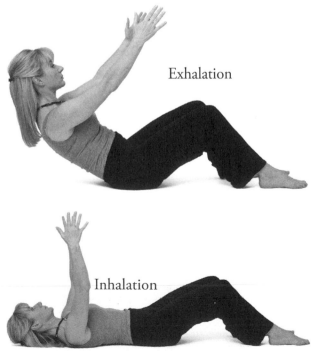

Exhalation

Inhalation

Effect
Strengthens the straight abdominal muscles and neck muscles.

Instructions
Lie on your back with your feet flat on the floor and knees bent. The feet are close to the buttocks hip width apart.

Exhaling
Raise the upper body slowly from the floor and stretch the arms straight upwards. Keep the neck long by drawing the breastbone towards the chin. Press the feet firmly to the floor.

Inhaling
Lower the upper body until the back of the head is about 5cm from the floor. The arms remain stretched upwards.

Repetition: × 10-12

Note: If the neck is uncomfortable, place the hands at the back of the head, exhaling to reduce the strain on the neck.

12. Variant of Jathara Parivritti

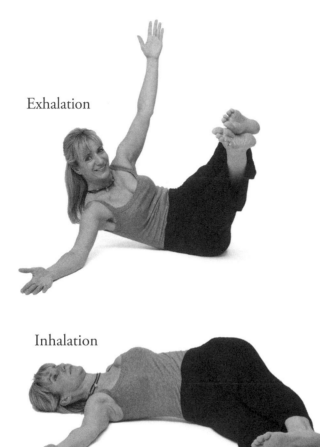

Exhalation

Inhalation

Effect
Strengthens the diagonal abdominal and deep-seated back extensor muscles. Mobilises the ribs and stretches the intercostal muscles.

Instructions
Lie on your back and stretch the arms to the sides at an angle of just less than 90 degrees, with the palms facing upwards. Move the knees to the right and stretch the legs out.

Exhaling
Raise the upper body and both legs from the floor at the same time and bring the stretched legs upwards vertically. Stretch the left arm towards the right side.

Inhaling
Lower both legs again without placing them on the floor. Then rest the upper body, head and left arm back on the floor. Press the backs of the hand into the floor to stabilise the position.

Repetition: 8 × each side

Note: If you suffer from back pain or slipped discs, this exercise is too harsh. Carry out the exercise with bent knees to reduce the strain on the lower back.

13. Siddhasana

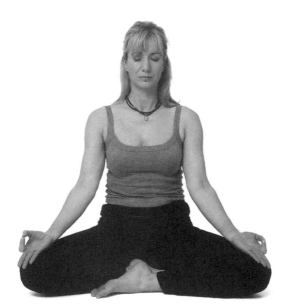

Effect
Straightens the spine and intensifies the inhalation.

Instructions
Come into a sitting position with crossed legs. Sit on a cushion to enable optimum alignment of the pelvis and spine.

Inhaling
In the first phase, breathe in from the collar bone to the breast bone and hold the breath briefly. In the second phase, inhale from the breastbone to the navel and hold the breath briefly. In the third phase, breathe down to the pelvic floor and hold the breath briefly.

Exhaling
Exhale very slowly and draw the abdominal wall in gently.

Repetition: 3-5 minutes

Note: If you feel short of breath, have breathing difficulties, high blood pressure or a heart complaint, this three-phase breathing exercise is not suitable. In this case, simply extend the inhalation a little and avoid over-straining.

Sidcways displacement of the spine / scoliosis (anatomy / theory)

Our spine forms the axis of the neck and body. It consists of 33 to 34 vertebrae, of which 24 move against one another. They are organised into 7 neck, 12 thoracic spine and 5 lumbar vertebrae, as well as associated discs, ligaments and muscles.

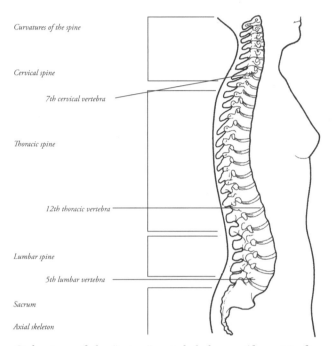

Curvatures of the spine

Cervical spine

7th cervical vertebra

Thoracic spine

12th thoracic vertebra

Lumbar spine

5th lumbar vertebra

Sacrum

Axial skeleton

Side view of the "spine" axial skeleton. (from Kraftsow, Kraftquelle Yoga) Fig. 13.

The coccyx consists of 3 to 5 reduced coccyx vertebrae (the remains of the tail of the vertebrate). From the side, four typical curvatures are apparent in the form of a double S-curve. The fixed (as it is ossified) sacral kyphosis and the three mobile sections lumbar lordosis, chest kyphosis and neck lordosis. Viewed from behind, the spine is like a pole. Deviations in the form of low-grade side displacements can be seen as individual within certain limits but not yet as indicative of disease (pathological).

The term "scoliosis" (Greek *skolios* = curved) primarily means a sideways bend of the spine, which can no longer be straightened out completely, but which is always associated with a twist in the vertebral body.

The causes are unknown for about 80 per cent of scoliosis cases (so-called idiopathic scoliosis).

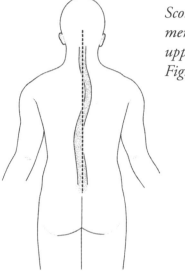

Scoliosis: sideways displacement in the lower and/or upper area of the back. Fig. 14.

With regard to the remaining 20 per cent, muscle, bone or other neurological diseases may be the cause. One reason may be a difference in the length of the legs, leading to misalignment of the pelvis. This then causes curvature of the spine or so-called functional scoliosis. Idiopathic scoliosis usually transpires at a period when the spine is subject to rapid growth. It therefore tends to be viewed as a growth deformity. It is usually discovered by chance in children and young people, and if left untreated, may lead to problems with the spine in advanced age, due to continuous incorrect loading. Internal organs such as the heart, lungs, kidneys, stomach and intestines may also be affected if scoliosis is not treated. In the early stages of scoliosis, therapeutic measures in particular, such as yoga therapy, physiotherapy, etc. are at the forefront. In the advanced stage, a corset or even an operation may be required. Early therapy often leads to good prospects for recovery. Depending on the locale, four different types of scoliosis may be encountered:

1. Thoracic scoliosis thoracic spine,

2. Lumbar scoliosis lumbar spine

3. Thoracic-lumbar scoliosis transferring from the chest to the lumbar spine,

4. Thoracic and lumbar scoliosis chest and lumbar spine.

Preconditions for a healthy spine

A well-functioning pelvis and trunk muscles with a spine that is axially well aligned. As scoliosis represents a displacement to the side, it is the muscles in the sides of the body, and the side pulls of the deep-seated back extensor muscles in particular, which are responsible. Well-aligned pelvis and leg statics are also important.

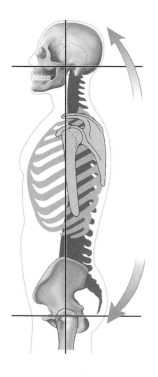

Extension of the spine through orientation and straightening of the pelvis and head. Fig. 15.

Muscular imbalances should be recognised and alleviated, for example, via yoga or other types of therapy. Regular exercise is important for this to succeed. Attention to the breathing also plays an important part here.

Objectives of yoga practice, particularly for scoliosis in the lower back

- Strength and mobility in the hips

- Mobility in the pelvis, iliosacral joint and groin area

- Redressing muscular imbalances in terms of pelvic statics

- Powerful and flexible leg and pelvis muscles (particularly buttock muscles and abductors)

- Strengthening and stretching in the abdominal and lower back muscles

- Optimum foot loading

Objectives of yoga practice, particularly for scoliosis in the upper back

- Redressing muscular imbalances in the shoulder, neck area and upper back,

- Mobility and flexibility in the thoracic spine area

- Strengthening and stretching the back and abdominal muscles

- Improved breathing and awareness of the breath

- Visualising axial length

- Mobilising the ribs

- Conscious breathing

Yoga programme for scoliosis of the lower back
Effects

- Stretches and strengthens the hip flexors

- Mobilises the iliosacral joints, lumbar spine and pelvis

- Lengthens and straightens the lower back

- Corrects misalignment of the pelvis by evening out muscular imbalances

- Stretches and strengthens the leg, buttock and back muscles

- Strengthens the diagonal abdominal and side buttock muscles

1. Variant of Jathara Parivritti

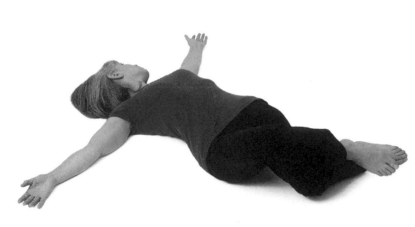

Effect
Mobilises the iliosacral joints and the pelvis. Stretches the outer buttocks and leg muscles.

Instructions
Lie on your back and place the feet hip width apart. Spread the arms out to the sides. Cross the right leg over the left one.

Exhaling
Let both knees sink to the right and turn the head to the left at the same time.

Repetition: Remain on each side for 6 breaths

Note: If you have backache, turning movements may cause pain. In this case, make a very slight turn outwards and ensure that your back remains in a natural curve.

2. Variant of Urdhva Prasarita Padasana

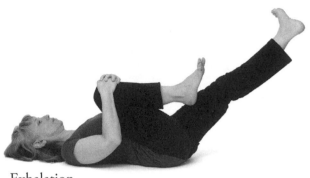

Exhalation

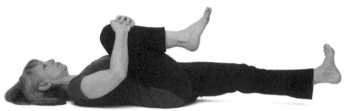

Inhalation

Effect
Stretches and strengthens the hip flexors and leg muscles. Balances misalignment of the pelvis.

Instructions
Remain on your back and pull the right knee towards the chest using both hands. The left leg is stretched out and the foot is turned 45 degrees outwards.

Exhaling
Raise the stretched leg around 1metre.

Inhaling
Let the left leg sink slowly without the foot touching the floor.

Repetition: 8-10 × each side

Note: This exercise should not cause pain in the lower back.

3. Postur Eka Pada Ustrasana

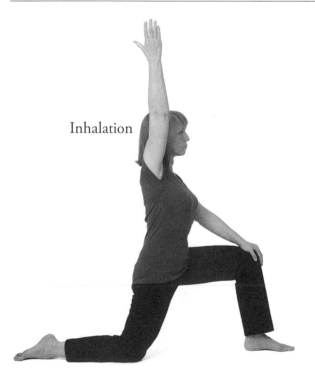

Inhalation

Effect
Stretches the hip flexors and enables asymmetrical extension of the spine.

Instructions
Come into a kneeling position and step the left foot forward. The knee and ankle are in alignment. Place both hands on the left thigh.

Inhaling
Raise the stretched right arm above the head. Extend the right groin area and the thigh.

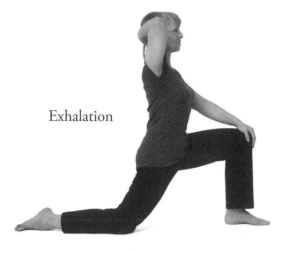

Exhalation

Exhaling

Move your centre of gravity further forward and intensify the stretch. At the same time bring the right hand to the back of the head.

Repetition: 8-10 × each side

Note: Avoid creating a large hollow in the lower back by raising the pubic bone slightly
Exhaling, and allowing the coccyx to lower when lengthening the lumbar spine. Take Note of which side of the groin contains more tension and repeat the exercise on this side twice more to even out muscular imbalances

4. Uttanasana

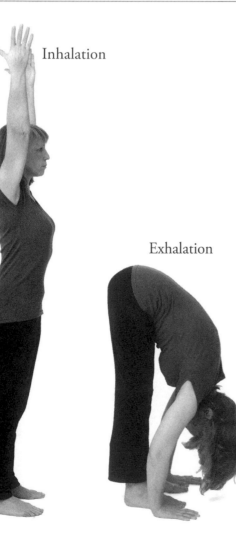

Inhalation

Exhalation

Effect

Stretches the lower back, leg and buttock muscles.

Instructions

Come into an upright standing position with the feet hip width apart.

Inhaling

Raise both stretched arms forwards above the head.

Exhaling

Bend forwards and place the hands on the floor. If you cannot stretch the legs this far, simply bend the knees to adapt the pose.

Repetition: × 8-10

Note: Forward bends can increase or even cause backache. If you have a sensitive lower back, go halfway into a forward bend and bend the knees even more.

5. Vinyasa Virabhadrasana and Parshva Uttanasana

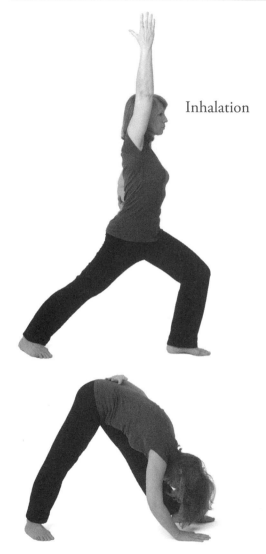

Inhalation

Exhalation

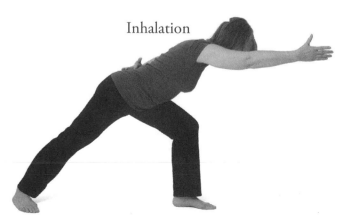

Inhalation

Effect
An asymmetrical stretch that strengthens the lower back, leg and buttock muscles.

Instructions
Come into the standing position and turn the right thigh outwards, so that the right foot is pointing out 45 degrees. Now take a long step forward with the left foot. Place the back of the left hand on the lower back.

Inhaling
Stretch the right arm forwards above the head and stretch the right side of the groin. Bend the left leg at the same time.

Exhaling
Come into a forward bend and stretch the left leg. Place the right hand on the floor.

Inhaling
Raise the upper body a little more than half way and stretch the right arm forwards. Bend the left leg again.

Repetition: 6 × each side

Note: In the forward bend, you can bend the front leg slightly if you are unable to stretch it. When coming up again, ensure you maintain a natural curvature in the lower back.

6. Variant of Ardha Parshva Uttanasana

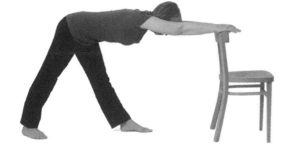

Effect
Asymmetrical stretch and extension of the lower back. Balances sideways abnormalities in the spine.

Instructions
Place a chair in front of you. Come into the same starting position as in the last exercise. Then bend forwards when

Exhaling and place the hands on the back of the chair. Stretch the spine and breathe in and out slowly. Extend the spine.

Repetition: Remain on each side for 6-8 breaths.

Note: An experienced yoga therapist can give you precise information in this posture for correcting muscular imbalances.

7. Chakravakasana

Exhalation

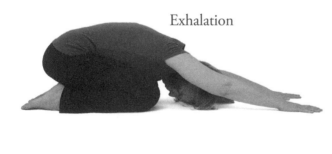

Effect
Stretches and mobilises the lower back and buttock area.

Instructions
Come on to all fours with the hands placed slightly in front of the shoulder joints.

Exhaling
Round the lower back and bring the buttocks backwards on to the heels. Stretch the lower back.

Inhalation

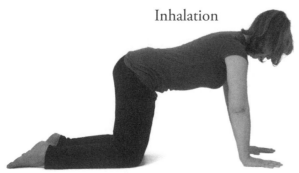

Inhaling
Come up again with the head and buttocks. Open the chest.

Repetition: × 8-10

8. Ardha Shalabhasana

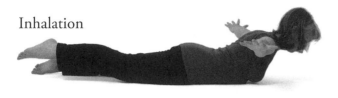

Inhalation

Exhalation

Effect
Asymmetrical strengthening of the lower back as well as the buttocks and the muscles at the back of the legs.

Instructions
Lie on your front. The head is turned to the side. The arms are placed next to the body.

Inhaling
Raise the head and chest, move both arms to the sides, and the right leg at the same time.

Exhaling
Lower the head and chest, both arms and the right leg back to the floor. Turn the head to alternate sides.

Repetition: 8-10 × each side

9. Apanasana

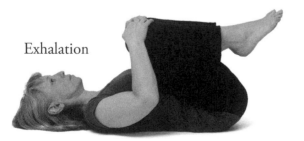

Exhalation

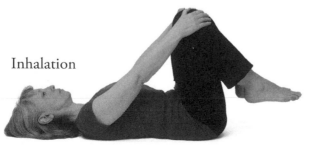

Inhalation

Effect
Stretches and relaxes the lower back

Instructions
Lie on your back with the feet on the floor and knees bent. Hold the knees with both hands.

Exhaling
Pull the knees towards the chest using both hands.

Inhaling
Move the knees forward until the arms are stretched out.

Repetition: 8-10 times

10. Exercise for the abdominal muscles

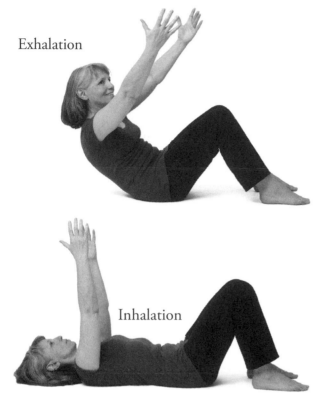

Exhalation

Inhalation

Effect
Strengthens the diagonal abdominal muscles and the neck.

Instructions
Lie on your back and place the feet close to the buttocks, hip width apart.

Exhaling
Raise the head and upper body from the floor and turn both to the right. At the same time stretch both arms upwards and to the right.

Inhaling
Lower the upper body and head again until they are 5cm from the floor.

Repetition: 8-10 × each side

Note: If you have neck problems, place one hand at the back of the head to reduce the strain on the neck.

11. Shavasana

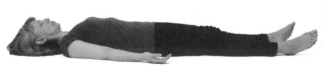

Effect
Relaxes the lower back. Extends the exhalation and calms the mind.

Instructions
Lying on your back, place the arms at the sides next to the body. Close your eyes. Breathe in deeply and out very slowly. After breathing out, activate the pelvic floor and pull the abdominal wall in gently. The inhalation should flow freely and the exhalation should be consciously extended.

Repetition: 3-5 minutes

Yoga programme for scoliosis in the upper back
Effects

- Rectifies muscular imbalances in the upper back and shoulder area

- Stretches and strengthens the back extensor muscles and shoulder blade muscles

- Improves movement and mobility in the thoracic spine

- Stretches and strengthens the intercostal and respiratory muscles

- Stretches and strengthens the neck muscles

- Stretches the spine to balance sideways displacement from scoliosis.

- Improved inhalation and energising effect

1. Dvipada Pitham

Inhalation

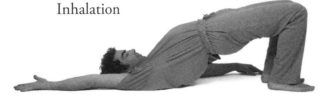

Exhalation

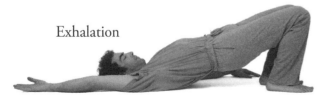

Effect
Opens the chest and one-sided extension and stretching in the upper back. Mobilises the thoracic spine.

Instructions
Lie on your back and place the feet hip width apart close to the buttocks. Place the arms at the sides of the body.

Inhaling
Raise the back and buttocks and stretch the right arm behind the head.

Exhaling
Place the upper back slowly back on the floor. The lower back and buttocks remain raised. The right arm stays behind the head.

Repetition: 8 × each side

Note: If you cannot stretch the arm, bend the elbow a little.

2. Variant of Chakravakasana

Inhalation

Exhalation

Effect
Strengthens the buttocks and lower back as well as asymmetrical stretching in the upper back.

Instructions
Come on to all fours and place the left hand about 10cm in front of the left shoulder joint. The right hand is directly under the right shoulder joint.

Inhaling
Stretch the right leg backwards and avoid clenching the lower back.

Exhaling
Bend the upper body forwards and place the right knee 10cm behind the left knee.

Repetition: 8 × each side

3. Eka Pada Ustrasana

Inhalation

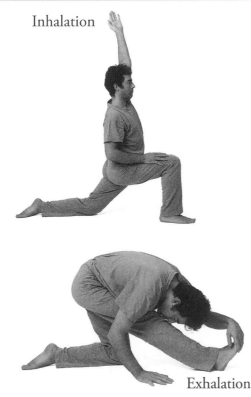

Exhalation

Effect
Asymmetrical stretching in the back, shoulder and buttock areas.

Instructions
Come into a kneeling position and step the right foot forwards on the floor. The knee and ankle should be in alignment.

Inhaling
Stretch the left arm above the head and extend the left thigh muscle.

Exhaling
Come into a forward bend, stretch the right leg and place the stomach on the right thigh. Move the left arm to the right foot and grip it. Keep the right hand on the floor to give support and stabilise the pose.

Repetition: 6 × each side, and then stay in the second position for 3 breaths.

4. Uttanasana

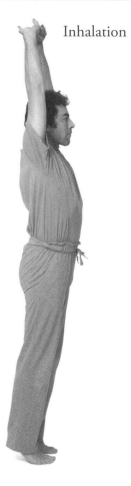

Inhalation

Effect
Stretches and strengthens the upper back and arm muscles.

Instructions
Come into an upright standing position with the feet hip width apart.

Inhaling
Raise the heels and stretch the arms forward above the head. The fingers are interlaced. Optimise the spinal extension by really stretching the abdominal muscles.

Exhaling
Lower the arms and place the heels back on the floor. Bring the buttocks backwards and bend slowly forwards. Place the palms on the floor. When Inhaling, come back up into the spinal extension by stretching the arms forward and emphasising the strengthening of the upper back.

Repetition: 8-10 times

Note: If your muscles at the back of the legs are shortened, you can bend the knee slightly when in the forward bend.

Exhalation

5. Ardha Parshva Uttanasana

Exhalation

Inhalation

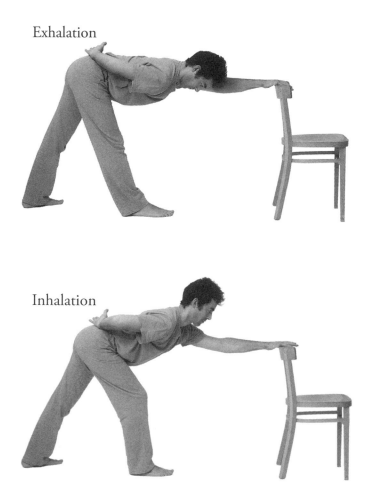

Effect
Asymmetrically stretches and strengthens the back extensor muscles, the sides of the ribs and the arm and shoulder muscles.

Instructions
Take a chair with a backrest or stand in front of a wall. Standing upright, turn the left leg outwards, so that the left foot is pointing out 45 degrees. Now take a large step backwards with the left foot. Place the hands on the back of the chair or on the wall.

Exhaling
Bend forwards and stretch the right leg and the spine. The left hand is placed on the back of the chair, and the back of the right hand is on the lower back. Change the distance of the chair with the front foot, so that the spine can be stretched as much as possible in the forward bend.

Inhaling
Bend the right leg and raise the head and chest a little. Ensure that the chest opens and the upper back stretches.

Repetition: 8 × each side

Note: An experienced yoga therapist can help you to correct any spine abnormality in this exercise. In my yoga therapy sessions, I measure the changes following the exercise using a scoliosis measuring device. I am always fascinated that sideways distortions of the spine can be corrected through regular yoga practice.

6. Variant of Prasarita Padottanasana

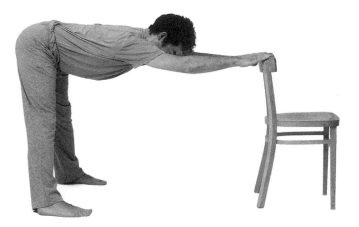

Effect
Stretches and strengthens the spine muscles. Balances sideways deviations through intensive stretching of the spine.

Instructions
Take a chair with a backrest or stand in front of a wall. Stand upright with both legs a little more than shoulder width apart. The hands are supported on the back of the chair or on the wall.

Exhaling
Come into the forward bend and place the fingers on the back of the chair. If your leg muscles are shortened you can bend the knees slightly.

Repetition: Remain in the position for 6-8 breaths.

7. Parshva Konasana

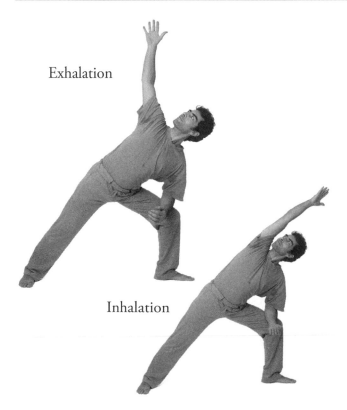

Exhalation

Inhalation

Effect
Mobilises the ribs and thoracic spine. Strengthens the shoulder and neck muscles.

Instructions
Stand upright with both legs considerably more than shoulder width apart. The left leg is turned outwards at an angle of 90 degrees.

Exhaling
Go into a left sideways bend and also bend the left leg, until the left knee is right above the ankle. Raise the right arm and turn the head upwards to the right, while the left lower arm is supported on the left thigh.

Inhaling
Move the right arm upwards towards the front of the body, while at the same time turning the head forwards towards the right hand. Stretch the sides of the ribs.

Repetition: 8 × each side

8. Vajrasana

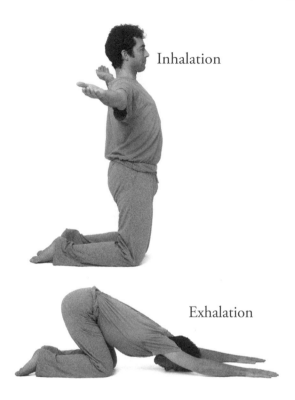

Inhalation

Exhalation

Effect
Opens the chest and stretches the upper back.

Instructions
Go into a kneeling position.

Inhaling
Raise the arms out to the sides and up to shoulder height. Open the chest.

Exhaling
Go into the forward bend with slightly bent knees, so that the buttocks remain in the air. Raise the outstretched arms in front of the head and on to the floor. Now push the breastbone towards the floor and stretch the upper back.

Repetition: 8-10 times

9. Vasisthasana

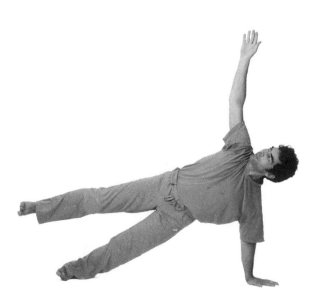

Effect
Strengthens the shoulder blades and arm muscles as well as the outer buttocks and lower back muscles.

Instructions
Exhaling, come off the knees into a sideways plank, by raising the knees from the floor and turning the stretched out legs to the left. Support yourself with your left hand. Stretch the right arm upwards and turn the head to the right to look at the right hand.

Inhaling
Raise the right leg about 40-60cm upwards with the hip and foot turned slightly inwards.

Repetition: Hold for 4-6 breaths

Note: Ensure that the elbows are not overstretched or turned inwards. If you have wrist problems you can support yourself on your lower arm. To simplify the exercise keep the right leg on the floor, which reduces the effort (see second photo).

10. Ardha Matsyendrasana

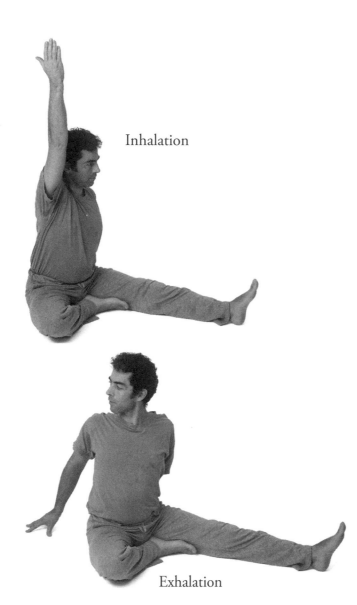

Inhalation

Exhalation

Effect

Mobilises the ribs and thoracic spine. Strengthens the middle and upper back between the shoulder blades.

Instructions

Sit in an upright position. Bend the right leg and lower the right knee downwards on to the floor. Place the right heel on the inside of the left thigh.

Inhaling

Stretch the right arm above the head. Raise the chin slightly. The left hand is placed on the floor to the left, next to the buttock.

Exhaling

Turn the body to the right and look over your right shoulder. Come on to the fingertips with the left hand to optimise the spinal extension and turn. Also support the right hand on its fingertips behind the buttocks.

Repetition: 6 × each side, then remain in the turn for 6 breaths.

Note: For the most Effective turn it is important to keep the spine straight. For many people this works better sitting on a cushion.

11. Vinyasa Dandasana and Paschimottanasana

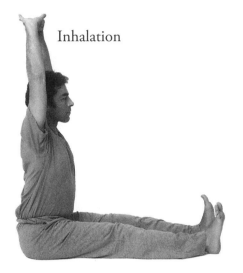
Inhalation

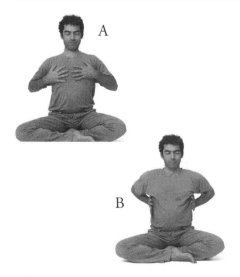
Exhalation

Effect
Stretches and strengthens the upper back and arms and straightens the neck.

Instructions
Sitting upright, stretch out both legs to the front. If you find it difficult to keep the pelvis straight, sit on a cushion.

Inhaling
Interlink the fingers and stretch the arms above the head. The palms are facing upwards.

Exhaling
Come into the forward bend with bent knees. Then place the hands at the back of the head and bring the elbows outwards next to the knee when bending forward, to give the upper back and shoulder area an optimum stretch.

Repetition: 8 times

12. Siddhasana

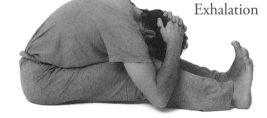
A

B

Effect
Stretches and strengthens the intercostal and respiratory muscles. Mobilises the thoracic spine and improves inhalation.

Instructions
Come into a comfortable sitting position. A. Place the hands on the upper ribs of the chest and take a long breath in. Then draw the ribs outwards using the fingers. After the inhalation hold the breath for 2-4 seconds and then breathe out slowly. Repeat 12 times. B. Now place the hands on the sides of the ribs. Draw the sides of the ribs backwards using the hands. After a long inhalation, hold the breath for 2-4 seconds and then exhale slowly. Repeat 12 times. Then place the hands on the knees and feel the uprightness of the spine and your inhalations.

Note: Find your own breathing rhythm, in which the breath flows long and steadily. You could try sitting on a cushion to keep the spine straight.

The upper back and opening up of the chest (anatomy / theory)

Our thoracic spine consists of 12 thoracic vertebral bodies that move against one another, the associated transverse and spinous processes and the articular processes. The vertebral bodies of the thoracic spine are more solid than those of the cervical spine and are part of the axial organs of our body. The bony chest (thorax) consists of the 12 thoracic vertebral bodies, the associated pairs of ribs and the breastbone (sternum). Ribs 1 to 7 sit directly at the front on the sternum; ribs 8 to 10 are connected together at the front by a cartilaginous ribcage; and ribs 11 and 12 are shorter and end unconnected in the abdominal wall. Between the ribs are the diagonal intercostal muscles, the so-called *intercostales externi* and *interni muscles*, which initiate the rise and fall of the ribs when exhaling and inhaling. The primary function of the chest is to protect the lungs and heart. The volume of the chest is decreased or increased due to the mobility of the ribs. The movement of the ribs thereby supports breathing, which takes place through muscular activity. The chest is separated from the abdominal area underneath by the diaphragm (main respiratory muscle).

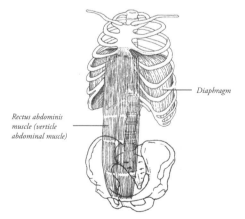

(from Kraftquelle Yoga, Vianova Verlag) Fig. 16.

Inhaling, the domes of the diaphragm move downwards towards the pelvis. The chest is integrated between the head, shoulder girdle and pelvis. The stabilising centre, the chest, is exposed to constant movement impulses from these three body sections

head/shoulder girdle and arms/pelvis, lumbar spine and legs.

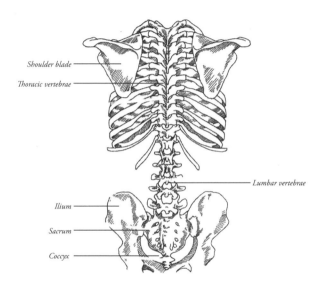

Bony connection shoulders/chest/pelvis(from Kraftquelle Yoga, Vianova Verlag) Fig. 17.

This requires so-called dynamic stabilisation. The breathing movements of the ribs also call for an activity that can be adapted.

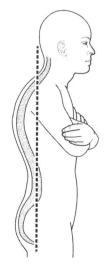

Kyphosis of the thoracic spine: noticeable curvature of the upper back. Fig. 18.

Where the shoulders are rounded and/or the back hunched, the breastbone sinks inwards and downwards and natural chest kyphosis is considerably increased. The movement of the ribs and thoracic spine decreases and becomes rigid and the breathing is significantly reduced. Cardiovascular activity is negatively affected. The inflexibility of the chest and the insufficiency of the respiratory muscles require an increased effort from the breathing mechanism. At the front of the body there is a shortening of the front muscle loops.

The causes may be very diverse

- habitual sitting positions where activities are primarily sedentary (*homo computerus*)

- cool poses adopted by many young people

- age-related kyphosisosteoporosis protective postures, such as are frequently found in basic depressive patterns

- systemic diseases of the thoracic spine, such as Scheuermann's Disease and Bekhterev's Disease

In the same way, a so-called *flat back* may affect the dynamics of breathing and chest mobility, thus becoming inflexible. A fixed, rigid chest lacks any dynamic adaptability. Both defects (hunched back and flat back) require compensatory mechanisms from the lumbar spine as well as from the cervical spine. They lead to chronic overloading of the cervical spine and /or lumbar spine, and the associated joints with their passive and active structures, and breathing is considerably reduced.

Different patterns of tension are dependent upon inner and outer effects. The relationship between emotional and physical processes is particularly clear. For example, with "breathing" any kind of activity / stress, whether physical or emotional, can directly affect the frequency and depth of breathing (particularly inhalation). Sayings such as

"to catch one's breath", "I held my breath", "paralysed by fear" or "I'm feeling hemmed in "are very significant.

In the example, the external "posture" tends to signify a sunken breastbone and kyphotic position of the thoracic spine

"I give in", "I don't want to stand out or attract attention" or "I'm holding back". A stiff back that is as straight as a die tends to be an expression of rigidity and fixity. It lacks any natural and dynamic adaptability. The heart chakra is assigned to this area.

Preconditions for a healthy thoracic spine

Due to everyday demands, e.g. sitting, many people suffer from a shortening of the front (ventral) muscle chain. This means that the area from the *tibialis ant. -> rectus femoris -> iliopsoas -> rectus abdominis -> to the front neck muscles* is shortened, and the back (dorsal) muscles are weakened. Due to chronic shortening of the front side and the back muscle chain that helps keep us erect, the disc structure is forced under pressure. The biomechanical displacement of the energies means that the increased output of energy in pressure is directed to the dynamic elements of the spine. Yoga therapy can help with this. The affected muscles are extended and strengthened, and it teaches awareness of the straightening and lengthening of the spine (body awareness), as well as consciousness of the breath. This means the spine is brought into movement (flexion, extension plus rotation and lateral flexion), the ribs and rib joints regain more room for movement, the muscle tone is regulated and the breathing can become deeper and more efficient.

Objectives of yoga therapy

- Stretching and opening the entire front muscle chain (hip flexors, abdominal and chest muscles and front neck muscles)

- Strengthening the whole back (dorsal) muscle chain

- Flexibility of the thoracic spine in all directions (particularly turning, bending to the side and stretching)

- Improving and training the mobility of the rib joints and the inhalation associated with this

- Integrating shoulder blade and arm muscles with the thorax

- Body awareness of the longitudinal axis / alignment of the spine

- Learning to maintain a natural pelvic position

- Strengthening the inhalation

- Natural, deep and relaxed flow of breath

- Promoting inner posture, openness and uprightness

Yoga programme for kyphosis / rounding of the back
Effects

- Stretches and strengthens the thigh muscles.

- Stretches the chest and shoulder blade muscles and the front side of the body

- Mobilises the thoracic spine and the ribs.

- Strengthens the arm and shoulder blade muscles.

- Strengthens the back and neck muscles.

- Opens and stretches the chest and rib muscles.

- Improves inhalation.

- Builds up energy.

- Opens up the heart and promotes self-awareness

1. Dvipada Pitham

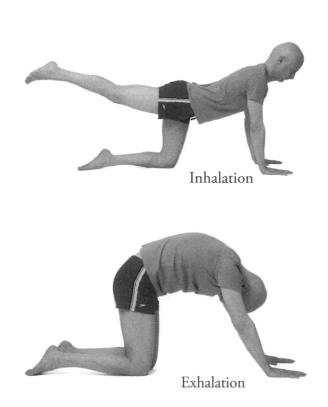

Inhalation

Exhalation

Effect
Stretches the chest muscles and strengthens the back muscles.

Instructions
Lie on your back and place the feet next to each other hip width apart.

Inhaling
Raise the buttocks off the floor and slide both arms along the floor to shoulder height. Open up the chest by raising the breastbone.

Exhaling
Lower the upper body and buttocks on to the floor and pull the knees towards the chest using both hands.

Repetition: × 8-10

2. Variant of Chakravakasana

Inhalation

Exhalation

Effect
Mobilises the thoracic spine and the ribs.

Instructions
Come on to all fours with the hips and knees in alignment. The hands are placed slightly in front of the shoulder joints for optimum mobilisation of the thoracic spine.

Inhaling
Raise and open the chest. At the same time stretch the right leg out behind you.

Exhaling
Place the right knee back on the floor and round the upper back like a cat arching its back. This mobiles the thoracic spine.

Repetition: 8-10 × each side

3. Eka Pada Ustrasana

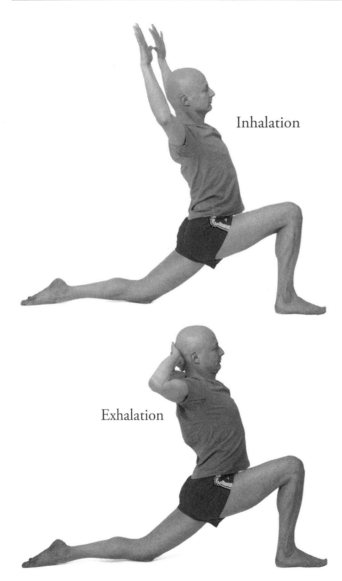

Inhalation

Exhalation

Effect
Stretches the chest and thigh muscles.

Instructions
Come into a kneeling position and step the right foot forward on the floor. The knee and ankle are in alignment.

Inhaling
Raise the bent arms to the sides above the head and stretch the chest.

Exhaling
Place both palms at the back of the head. At the same time push the left side of the groin forwards and stretch the left thigh muscles.

Repetition: 8-10 × each side

Note: Exhaling, raise the breastbone slightly to optimise the opening of the chest. Raise the pubic bone upwards slightly to avoid clenching in the lower back.

4. Vinyasa Tadasana and Ardha Utkatasana

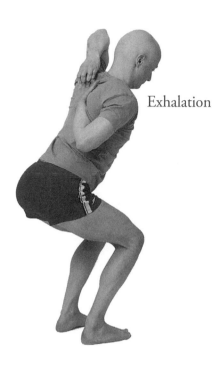

Exhalation

Effect
Stretches the shoulder blade muscles and the side rib muscles. Strengthens the muscles of the upper arm.

Instructions
Come into an upright standing position with the feet hip width apart. Take the back of the right hand behind the back and upwards to the left shoulder blade. Stretch the left arm upwards and over the shoulder. Now move the fingers together. You may be able to interlock the fingers. The stretch should not be painful.

Exhaling
Come slowly into a semi-squat and bring the buttocks backwards. Move the knees forward but not too far (overloading). Avoid splaying the knees or feet inwards or outwards. The spine remains as stretched as possible.

Inhaling
Come out of the squat and raise the heels from the floor.

Repetition: 8 × each side

Note: If you have shortened arms and shoulder blade muscles, the fingers may not grip one another. In this case, adapt the exercise by leaving the hands apart and avoiding too strong a stretch.

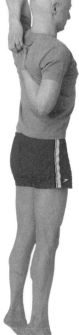

Inhalation

5. Vinyasa Virabhadhrasana and Utthita Trikonasana

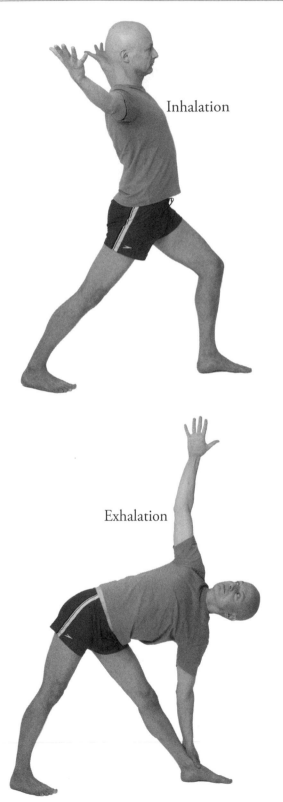

Inhalation

Exhalation

Effect
Opens the chest and rib muscles. Mobilises the thoracic spine and strengthens the neck.

Instructions
From the upright standing position, turn the right leg out so that the right foot is pointing 45 degrees outwards. Now take a large step forward with the left foot and bend the left leg.

Inhaling
Stretch both arms out to the sides at shoulder height and expand the chest by raising the breastbone. The palms are facing upwards and the shoulder blades remain relaxed.

Exhaling
Come into a forward bend with a stretched spine and then turn the spine to the right. Move the right hand and head upwards vertically. Place the left hand on the left shin.

Repetition: 6 × each side, then remain in the second position for 3 breaths.

Note: To avoid turning the head too sharply upwards, look downwards towards the front foot.

6. Vinyasa Virabhdrasana and Parshva Uttanasana

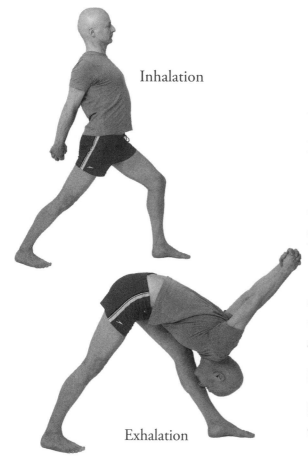

Inhalation

Exhalation

Effect
Stretches the chest and strengthens the arm and shoulder girdle muscles.

Instructions
The same starting position as in the last exercise. However, make the step forward somewhat longer and place the arms behind the back with the fingers interlocked.

Inhaling
Open the chest by raising the breastbone and stretching the arms actively away from the shoulders. After Inhaling hold the breath for 2-4 seconds.

Exhaling
Go into the forward bend and stretch the left leg. At the same time, take the arms back and stretch the arms away from the shoulders.

Repetition: 8 × each side

Note: Move the breastbone forwards and upwards at the same time when you inhale, to achieve optimum opening of the chest.

7. Natarajasana

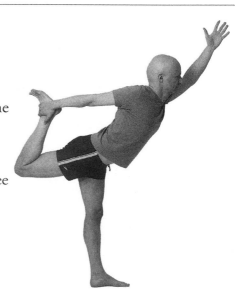

Effect
Balances and strengthens the leg muscles and opens the chest.

Instructions
In the upright standing position, bend the right knee backwards and hold the front of the right foot behind the body using both hands.

Exhaling
Move the upper body forward, keeping the back long, and pull the right knee backwards and up.

Inhaling: Stretch the left arm forwards and upwards.

Repetition: Hold on each side for 6 breaths.

Note: Avoid clenching the lower back in this exercise by slightly raising the pubic bone towards the navel.

8. Vajrasana

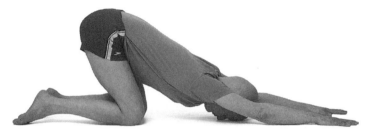

Effect
Extends the thoracic spine and stretches the under-arms.

Instructions
Come on to all fours. The knee and ankle are in alignment. The hands are placed in front of the shoulder joints. Keep the knees a little more than hip width apart.

Exhaling
Move the buttocks backwards and upwards, so that the thighs are vertical in the forward bend. Place the forehead on the floor and stretch the thoracic spine by allowing the breastbone to sink on the exhalation.

Repetition: Remain for 6-8 breaths.

9. Ustrasana

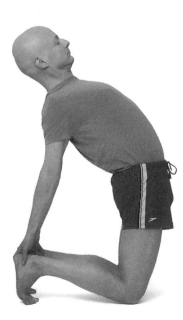

Effect
Opens the chest and strengthens the neck and back muscles.

Instructions
Come into a kneeling position.

Exhaling
Raise the breastbone and bring the upper body back carefully into a backward bend. Take the hands slowly towards the ankles. Keep the neck long. Avoid clenching in the neck and lower back.

Repetition: Remain for 3-6 breaths

Note: This position is too intense if you have back and neck problems. If this is the case, do the exercise from a squat position with the support of your hands.

10. Paschimottanasana

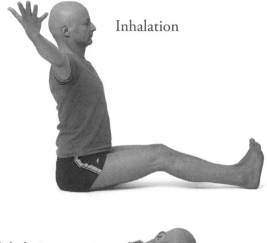

Inhalation

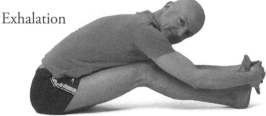

Exhalation

Effect
Gently stretches the lower back. Relaxes the neck and shoulders.

Instructions
Sit in an upright position and bend the knees slightly.

Inhaling
Raise both arms to the sides up to shoulder height and the breastbone slightly at the same time.

Exhaling
Come into a gentle forward bend with very bent knees. Bring the chest to the thighs and the palms to the balls of the feet. Then turn the head alternately to the right and left sides.

Repetition: × 8-10

Note: If you find it difficult to keep the pelvis and spine straight, sit on a cushion.

11. Bharadvajasana

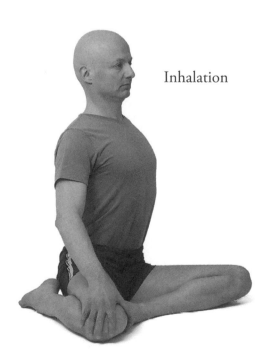

Inhalation

Effect
Stretches the chest. Intensive mobilisation of the thoracic spine and ribs. Strengthens the deep-seated back extensor muscles and neck muscles.

Instructions
Remain in an upright sitting position and bring the right leg backwards with the knee bent. Place the back of the right foot to the side, next to the right buttock. The left leg is bent with the knee outwards to the left and the left sole of the foot on the inside of the right thigh. Now place the right hand on the right knee and bring the fingertips of the left hand behind the left hip.

Inhaling
Straighten the pelvis and stretch the spine along its length.

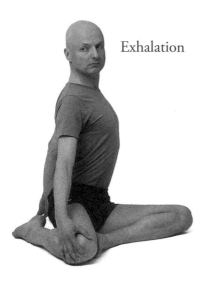

Exhalation

Exhaling

Move the left shoulder back and to the left and at the same time turn the head right to the opposite side.

Repetition: Remain for 8 breaths on each side in the second rotation.

Note: Intensify the opening of the chest and optimise the spiral twist movement when Exhaling by stretching the right side of the body and ribs. When Inhaling, activate the pelvic floor and straighten the spine. Raise the right sitting bone slightly off the floor to optimise the stretch and rotation.

12. Siddhasana

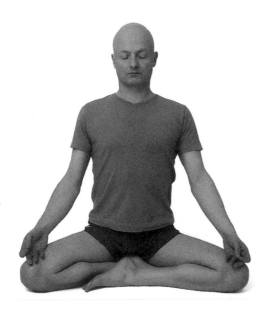

Effect

Lengthens the inhalation and extends the fullness of the breath. Increases the intake of oxygen and builds up energy.

Instructions

Come into a comfortable sitting position. Inhale from the upper ribs to the breastbone. Hold the breath after Inhaling. Continue the breaths until the breath reaches the pelvic floor. Exhale again slowly and draw in the abdominal wall gently at the same time.

Breathing rhythm

Inhalation: 3 seconds (to the breastbone),
2 second pause
Inhalation: 3 seconds (to the pelvic floor)
Exhalation: 8 seconds
Repetition: × 6

Inhalation: 4 seconds (to the breastbone),
2 second pause
Inhalation: 4 seconds (to the pelvic floor)
Exhalation: 10 seconds
Repetition: × 6

Inhalation: 5 seconds (to the breastbone), 2 second pause
Inhalation: 5 seconds (to the pelvic floor)
Exhalation: 10 seconds
Repetition: × 6

Inhalation: 3 seconds (to the breastbone),2 second pause
Inhalation: 3 seconds (to the pelvic floor)
Exhalation: 8 seconds
Repetition: × 6

Observe whether you feel comfortable doing this and adapt the rhythm of the breath to your current state.

Note:

Do not force the breath in any way and avoid too much pressure in the head and neck area. If you have high blood pressure, migraine or a heart complaint, do not hold the breath after the inhalation. Respect your limits.

Relaxed shoulders and a free neck (anatomy / theory)

The shoulder girdle connects the arms with the upper spine, just as the pelvic girdle joins the legs to the lower spine. As the shoulder joint, in contrast to other joints (e.g. the hip joint), is primarily stabilised by the muscles, this enables the greatest mobility and flexibility on the one hand, but it also allows less stability on the other hand. Therefore, it can also mean greater susceptibility to injuries and problems. The arms and body are connected together by the smooth interplay of several joints.

These joints are

- The shoulder joint (humeroscapular joint) and the subacromial space

- The joint connection from the collar bone to the acromial joint and from the collar bone to the breastbone (sternoclavicular joint) and the sliding plane of the shoulder blade at the chest (scapulothoracic sliding plane)

- For the arm move to within its full range, the mobility of the ribs and a flexible and upright spine are important, along with the "shoulder" joint complex

The cervical spine is the most mobile part of the spine. It consists of seven smaller, delicate vertebrae with wide transverse processes, through the opening of which the *arteria vertebralis* passes. The two upper neck vertebrae (atlas and axis) differ considerably from the others. The first and topmost cervical vertebral body, the atlas, carries the head and has no vertebral bodies. It is rather like a ring with two strong side areas (*massae lateralis*) with joint surfaces lying above and below. The upper joint surfaces are connected to the base of the cranium and the lower ones are connected to the second cervical vertebral body, the axis. The second cervical vertebra has a tooth-shaped extension (*dens axis*) on its upper part. This *dens* is connected as a pivot joint with the atlas above it. The result is very good rotational capability. The seventh cervical vertebral body is also called the *vertebra prominens*, as its spinous process protrudes the furthest back. It is easily palpable and offers a good reference point for cervicothoracic junction, (the area where the neck and thoracic spine meet). The discs are located between the neck vertebrae as they are in the rest of the spine. The cervical spine is supported by the surface neck muscles and upper back muscles, as well as by the deep-seated autochthonous back muscles and several important ligamentous structures. Their process is similar to a gentle curvature (lordosis), like that of the lumbar spine.

The junction of the neck and thoracic spine and the musculoskeletal system of the shoulder girdle represents a very complex area from the perspective of biomechanics.

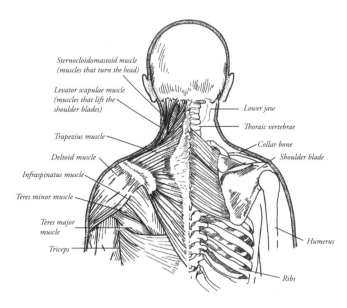

Sternocloidomastoid muscle (muscles that turn the head)

Levator scapulae muscle (muscles that lift the shoulder blades)

Trapezius muscle

Deltoid muscle

Infraspinatus muscle

Teres minor muscle

Teres major muscle

Triceps

Lower jaw

Thoraic vertebrae

Collar bone

Shoulder blade

Humerus

Ribs

(from Kraftquelle Yoga, Vianova Verlag) Fig. 19.

To give a rough overview, it is a good idea to look at the surface muscles in this region:

From the front, it is the major chest muscles (*pectoralis major*) and the shoulder cap muscles (*deltoideus*) that catch our attention first. Deep-seated and not visible are the small chest muscles (*pectoralis minor*).

The muscles that connect the chest and cervical spine, include the sternocleidomastoids and the scalene muscles.

The muscles that connect the body with the arms include the *biceps brachii*, the *coracobrachialis* and, from behind, the *triceps brachii*.

When viewed from the back, the following surface layer of muscles is visible, consisting of the *trapezius*, *teres major, latissimus dorsi* and *deltoideus*. Covered by the upper part of the trapezius muscles are the shoulder blade lifters (*levator scapulae*) and the shoulder blade connecters, the so-called rhombus-shaped muscles (rhomboidei, major and minor) and the rotator sleeve (*supraspinatus* and *infraspinatus, teres minor* and *subscapularis*).

Even deeper and covered by the muscles mentioned above, are the autochthonous back muscles close to the spine (spinotransversal system, intertransversal system and transversospinal system). In general, we can say that they are sub-divided into a medium and deep-seated layer and serve to keep the (cervical) spine erect, rotate it and incline it to the side. They cannot be controlled in isolation.

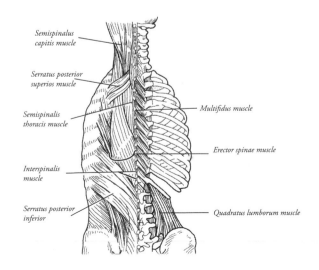

Semispinalus capitis muscle

Serratus posterior superios muscle

Semispinalis thoracis muscle

Interspinalis muscle

Serratus posterior inferior

Multifidus muscle

Erector spinae muscle

Quadratus lumborum muscle

(from KraftquelleYoga, Vianova Verlag) Fig. 20.

Expressions such as "he has some neck", "to get it in the neck" and "carrying the weight of the world on your shoulders" are well-known. It is also clear here how the inner attitude affects the outer. In psychosomatics, the neck vertebrae also stand for communication, self-expression and the extent to which one is open to life. The throat chakra is allocated to the cervical spine.

Preconditions for a relaxed shoulder and neck area

Due to the many repetitive movement processes and one-sided static body positions (e.g. sitting at the computer without any breaks, or long hours of driving a vehicle without any stops), the shoulder girdle and cervical spine are nearly always problem areas, with functional problems, protective postures and pain. Complaints originating in the cervical spine often radiate out into the shoulder and arm region.

Those affected often report that they feel internal tension, a burning and pulling pain in the neck region, which extends from the back of the head to the shoulder blades.

The functional inter-relationship (muscle chain, muscle loops and movement axes) from the pelvis, lumbar spine, thoracic spine and cervical spine, should always be considered. Due to lack of movement, the muscles are subject to fixed shortening, resulting in weakness. The muscles therefore need to be extended and strengthened (e.g. with yoga) so that they have the opportunity to work in an optimum way. The pressure on the joints and discs is optimised, the neck can experience space and length once again, the head is free to move and the arms and shoulder girdle can unfold in their full mobility, stability and strength and vascular and nerve paths can flow afresh. This reinstates the profile required for the shoulder and neck.

Regularly practising your own yoga programme will help you achieve an inner and outer body consciousness. This teaches you to to be automatically aware of the natural, healthy alignment of the spine and joints, particularly the organisation of the shoulder girdle, the cervicothoracic junction and the position of the head.

Objectives in yoga therapy

- Releasing and extending tense neck and shoulder muscles

- Mobilising the cervical spine and the junction with the thoracic spine and shoulder girdle

- Stretching the chest and front neck muscles

- Mobilising and strengthening the shoulder blade muscles

- Toning (strengthening) the neck, shoulder and arm muscles

- Teaching body awareness, (alignment of the spine, pelvis and head joints, relaxing the shoulder girdle, etc.)

- Relaxing the jaw and masticatory muscles

- Mobilising the chest

- Awareness of the breath; more relaxed and deeper flow of the breath

Yoga programme for relaxed shoulders and a free neck

Effects

- Mobilises the shoulder joints and cervical spine.

- Stretches and strengthens the neck muscles.

- Improves mobility and blood flow in the neck.

- Extends and strengthens the shoulder blade muscles.

- Stretches the large and small chest muscles.

- Improves mobility in the upper back and ribs.

- Strengthens the muscles between the shoulder blades and the upper arm muscles.

- Encourages awareness of optimum arm movement and head position.

- Calms the mind and nervous system using sounds.

- Relaxes the jaw and neck area.

1. Variant of Shavasana

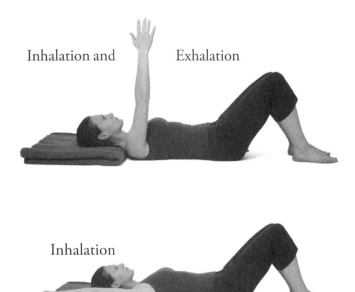

Inhalation and   Exhalation

Inhalation

Effect
Relaxes the shoulder blade muscles and encourages optimum positioning of the shoulders

Instructions
Lie on your back with knees bent and position the feet hip width apart. Place a folded blanket underneath the head

Inhaling
Raise the right arm vertically.

Exhaling
Let the right shoulder blade fall to the floor and at the same time relaxthe shoulder muscles.

Inhaling
Stretch the right arm behind the head.

Exhaling
Raise the right arm vertically and bring it back on to the floor.

Repetition: 8-10 × each side

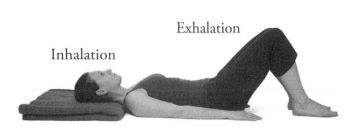

Exhalation

Inhalation

2. Variant of Shavasana

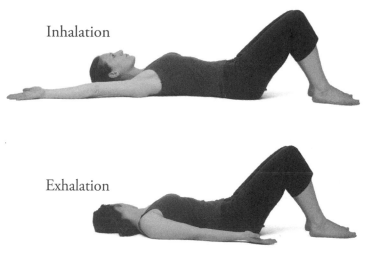

Inhalation

Exhalation

Effect
Mobilises the neck and ribs and stretches the sides.

Instructions
Remain lying on your back and place the feet close to the buttocks, hip width apart.

Inhaling
Slide the right arm sideways along the floor above the head.

Exhaling
Move the right arm back along the floor and turn the head to the left at the same time.

Repetition: 8 × each side

Note: If you have a sensitive neck, turn the head only as far as is comfortable.

3. Variant of Chakravakasana

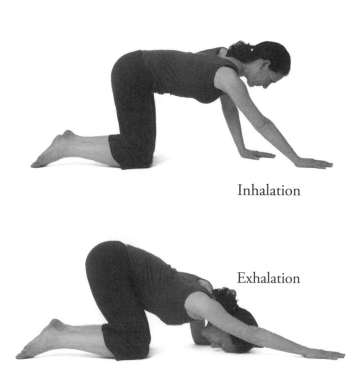

Inhalation

Exhalation

Effect
Stretches the arm and shoulder blade muscles. Extends the upper back.

Instructions
Come on to all fours. The hips and knees are in alignment. The hands are placed slightly in front of the shoulder joints. Place the right hand about 10cm further forward.

Inhaling
Open and mobilise the chest.

Exhaling
Move the pelvis backwards slightly, so that the bent left lower arm is lying on the floor. Place the forehead on the floor if possible. The buttocks remain in the air.

Repetition: 8-10 × each side

4. Uttanasana

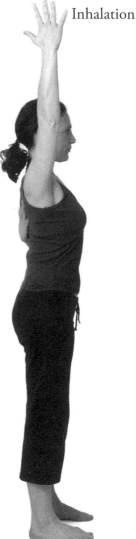

Inhalation

Effect
Stretches the neck, shoulder and arm muscles. Mobilises the neck and shoulder blades.

Instructions
Come into an upright standing position with the feet hip width apart. Bring the back of the left hand to the right shoulder blade.

Inhaling
Stretch the right arm above the head.

Exhaling
Come into the forward bend with the right arm stretched downwards and turn the head to the right, while moving the left shoulder backwards and upwards.

Inhaling
Come back up into the starting position with the back extended.

Repetition: 8 × each side

Note: If you are not very mobile in the lower back, you can bend the knee slightly in the forward bend.

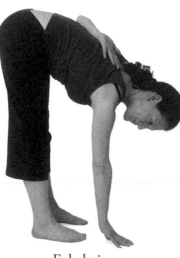

Exhalation

5. Ardha Utkatasana and Uttanasana

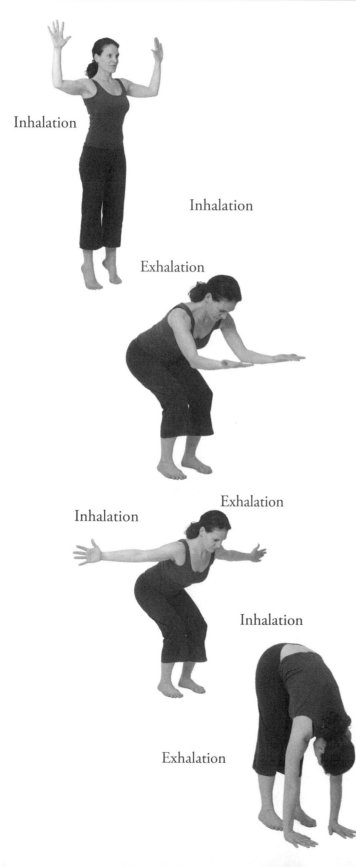

Inhalation

Inhalation

Exhalation

Exhalation

Inhalation

Inhalation

Exhalation

Effect
Strengthens the muscles between the shoulder blades and strengthens the thigh muscles.

Instructions
Come into an upright standing position with the feet hip width apart.

Inhaling
Raise both arms out to the sides to shoulder height with the forearms pointing up vertically. At the same time, raise the heels off the floor.

Exhaling
Bring the heels on to the floor. Bend the knee and go into a squat. Stretch out the arms in front of the body with the palms upwards.

Inhaling
Stretch the arms out to the sides.

Exhaling
Stretch the legs and come into the forward bend. Place the hands on the floor and stretch the lower back.

Repetition: × 6

Note: Do not move the knee too far forward in the squat. The weight of the feet is distributed across three points. You can also adapt the forward bend by bending the knee slightly.

6. Virabhadrasana and Utthita Trikonasana

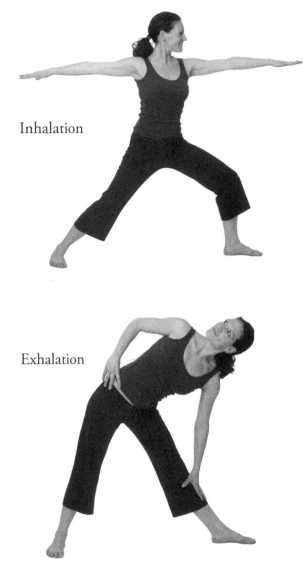

Inhalation

Exhalation

Effect
Strengthens the upper arm and the muscles that turn the head. Encourages mobility of the ribs, thoracic spine and neck.

Instructions
In the upright standing position, turn the right leg out, so that the right foot is pointing 45 degrees outwards. Now take a large step forward with the left foot and bend the left leg.

Inhaling
Raise both arms to the sides until they are a little below the height of the shoulder joints.

Exhaling
Bend your upper body horizontally to the left and forwards. Stretch the left leg and turn the body and the head upwards and to the right. Place the left hand on the shin and the right hand on the right side of the pelvis.

Repetition: 8-10 × each side

Note: If you have neck problems, move the head upwards only slightly. Avoid hoisting up the shoulder blades and overstretching the elbows in the first position.

7. Virabhadrasana and Parshva Uttanasana

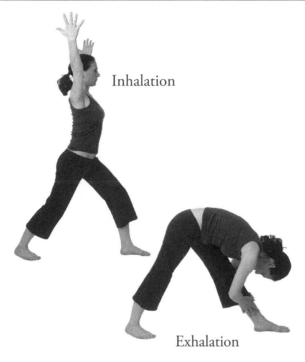

Inhalation

Exhalation

Effect
Stretches the chest and rib muscles. Strengthens the wide back and shoulder blade muscles.

Instructions
The same starting position as before, with the left foot placed in front and the left leg bent.

Inhaling
Stretch both arms out to the sides and move them upwards wide open. Relax and lower the shoulders and open the chest.

Exhaling
Come into a half forward bend and stretch the left leg. Place both hands on the left shin. Move both shoulder blades outwards and round the upper back.

Repetition: 8-10 × each side

8. Variant of Chakravakasana

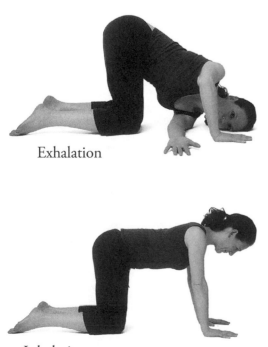

Exhalation

Inhalation

Effect
Stretches the shoulder blades and neck muscles. Mobilises the upper back and neck.

Instructions
Come on to all fours. The hips and knees are in alignment. The hands are placed slightly in front of the shoulder joints.

Exhaling
Slide the left arm along the floor to the right and under the right arm and also turn the head to the right. At the same time turn the upper body to the right and forwards.

Inhaling
Come back on to all fours, by stretching the left arm again and raising the upper body.

Repetition: 6-8 × each side

Note: You may need to use a cushion to rest the head more easily to the side.

9. Dvipada Pitham

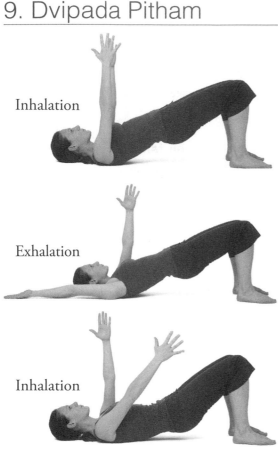

Inhalation

Exhalation

Inhalation

Effect
Releases tension between the shoulder blades. Stretches the neck. Mobilises the upper thoracic spine.

Instructions
Lie on your back and place the feet close to the buttocks, hip width apart.

Inhaling
lift the pelvis off the floor and raise both arms upwards vertically.

Exhaling
Move the right arm forward and place the upper back slowly on the floor again disc by disc.

Inhaling
Move the right arm backward and raise the upper back again. Open the chest.

Repetition: 8-10 × each side

10. Jathara Parivritti

Effect
Mobility in the neck, ribs and spine. Stretches the neck and chest muscles.

Instructions
Remain lying on your back with the knees bent. Move the arms out to the sides away from the body at a 90 degree angle. Exhaling, let both knees sink to the right.

Inhaling
Raise the left arm vertically and let the left shoulder blade rest on the floor.

Exhaling
Bring the left arm back to the floor and turn the head to the left.

Repetition: 8-10 × each side

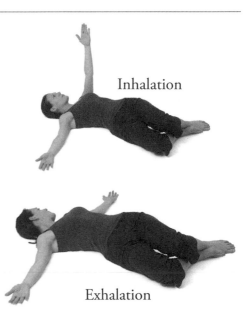

Inhalation

Exhalation

Note: If you have neck problems, turn the head very carefully. The exercise should not cause any pain whatsoever.

11. Vajrasana

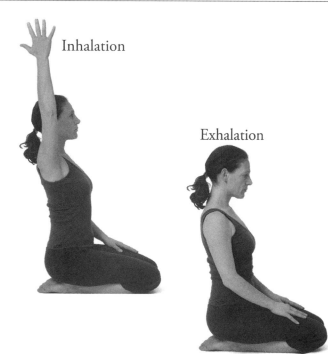

Inhalation

Exhalation

Effect
Relaxes the jaw and neck area. Calms the mind and the nervous system.

Instructions
Come into the squat. If you find this position difficult, place a cushion under the buttocks.

Inhaling
Stretch the right arm above the head. At the same time raise the head a little.

Exhaling
Hum a deep "om". Lower the right arm and move the head downwards a little.

Repetition: 6 × each side

12. Shavasana

Effect
Deep relaxation of the neck and mind.

Instructions
Lie on your back. Place the arms at the sides of the body with the palms facing upwards. The legs are slightly open and the feet pointing outwards. The eyes are closed. Place a folded blanket under the back of the head and neck.

Inhaling
Inhale gently through the nose.

Exhaling
Exhale through the open mouth and hum "om" in your mind. Relax the neck and shoulder blade muscles.

Repetition: 2-3 minutes and then remain still

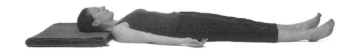

Yoga programme for strong shoulders and a strong neck

Effects

- Strengthens the shoulder blade muscles and stabilises the shoulder blades

- Strengthens the sternocleidomastoid muscles that turn the head, and the neck muscles

- More mobility in the upper back, shoulders and neck area

- Strengthens the large and side buttock muscles

- Stretches the chest and the sides of the ribs

- Strengthens the different arm muscles and the *serratus* muscles

- Energising effect due to improved inhalation capacity

1. Dvipada Pitham

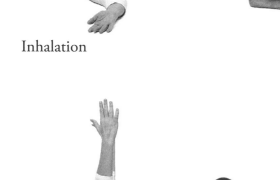

Inhalation

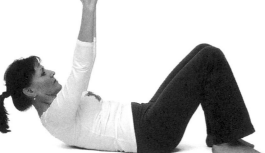

Exhalation

Effect

Opens the chest as well as stretching and strengthening the abdominal and neck muscles.

Instructions

Lie on your back and place the feet close to the buttocks, hip width apart.

Inhaling

Raise the buttocks from the floor and take both arms out to the sides. Concentrate on widening the chest.

Exhaling

Place the lower back and buttocks back on the floor and raise the head and upper body. Draw both arms upwards.

Repetition: × 8-10

Note: If you have a sensitive neck, raising the head may cause too much stress. In this case, keep the back of the head and the upper body on the floor when exhaling.

2. Variant of Chakravakasana

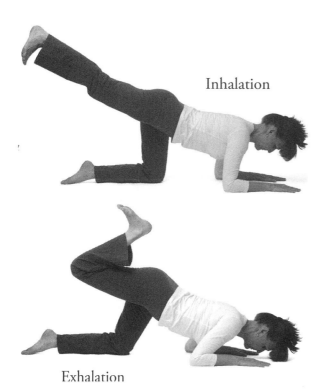

Inhalation

Exhalation

Effect
Strengthens the arm, shoulder blade, leg and buttock muscles.

Instructions
Come on to all fours. Place the forearms on the floor.

Inhaling
Stretch the right leg backwards without curving the spine. The right heel is pushed backwards and the toes move forwards.

Exhaling
Come towards the floor with the upper body. At the same time bend the right leg and both arms, with the elbows remaining close to the body. Take care to work with the shoulders and do not let the shoulders hang down.

Repetition: 8-10 × each side

Note: Ensure that the pelvis held horizontally and does not jut out. Activate the pelvic floor and the abdominal muscles to stabilise the pelvis.

3. Variant of Chakravakasana

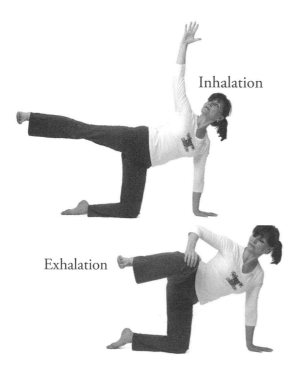

Inhalation

Exhalation

Effect
Strengthens the arm, shoulder and serratus muscles. Stabilises the shoulder blades.

Instructions
Come on to all fours. The hands are placed directly underneath the shoulder joints.

Inhaling
Raise the right arm and at the same time move the right, outwards rotated leg upwards. Turn the body, pelvis and head upwards to the right.

Exhaling
Bend the right leg and bring the knee out horizontally to hip height. Lower the right arm and place the right hand on the right knee.

Repetition: 8-10 × each side

4. Vinyasa Tadasana and Uttanasana

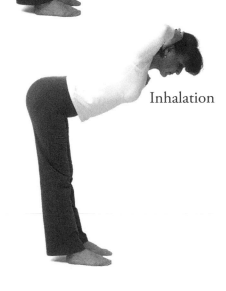

Inhalation

Exhalation

Inhalation

Effect
Strengthens the shoulder blades and neck muscles as well as the back extensor muscles.

Instructions
Come into an upright standing position with the feet hip width apart.

Inhaling
Raise the heels and stretch the arms above the head. Interlock the fingers with the palms facing upwards.

Exhaling
Interlink the hands behind the head and bend your upper body forwards in a front bend.

Inhaling
Come upwards with your upper body into a half forward bend and move the elbows wide apart. Bring both shoulder blades in towards one another.

Repetition: × 6

Note: If you cannot stretch the legs, bend the knee slightly. If you have a sensitive lower back, bend the knees and go only as far as is comfortable in the forward bend

5. Vinyasa Virabdhrasana and Utthita Trikonasana

Inhalation

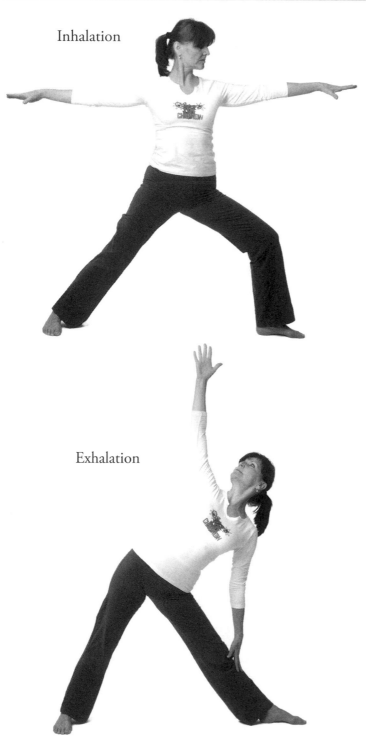

Exhalation

Effect
Strengthens the arm and shoulder muscles as well as the sternocleidomastoid muscles that move the head. Mobilises the thoracic spine and stretches one side of the sternocleidomastoid muscles.

Instructions
Take a large step forwards with the left leg. The back right foot is rotated outwards at 90 degrees.

Inhaling
Bend the left knee in alignment with the ankle and raise both arms to the side at shoulder height. Splay the fingers and move the head to look towards the left hand.

Exhaling
Bend the upper body forward with outstretched arms and then turn the upper body to the right. Place the left hand on the left shin and turn the head upwards towards the right hand.

Repetition: 6 × each side, then remain in the second position for 3 breaths.

Note: If you have a sensitive neck, you can also turn the head downwards to the front foot turn so that the neck is not strained.

6. Utthita Trikonasana

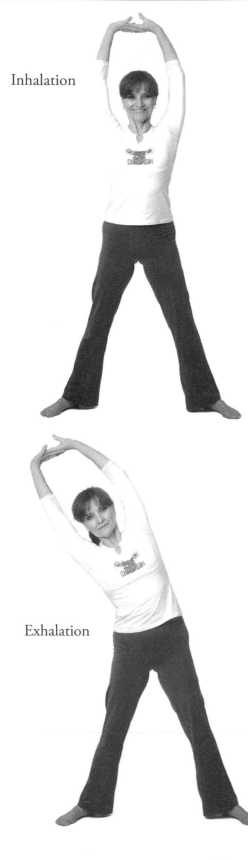

Inhalation

Exhalation

Effect

Opens the intercostal muscles and mobilises the upper back. Stretches the chest. Strengthens the arm and shoulder blade muscles.

Instructions

Stand with legs splayed more than shoulder width apart. Both legs are rotated slightly outwards and the feet are pointed outwards a little.

Inhaling

Interlink the fingers together and stretch the arms above the head.

Exhaling

Move your upper body towards the right into a side bend and open the sides of the ribs and the left side of the chest. Feel the stretch from the left hips into the hand.

Repetition: 8 × each side

Note: If you have a sensitive lower back, you should only carry out a slight sideways bend. Avoid clenching the side towards which you are bending. It is better to stretch both sides of the trunk at the same time.

7. Adho Mukha Svanasana

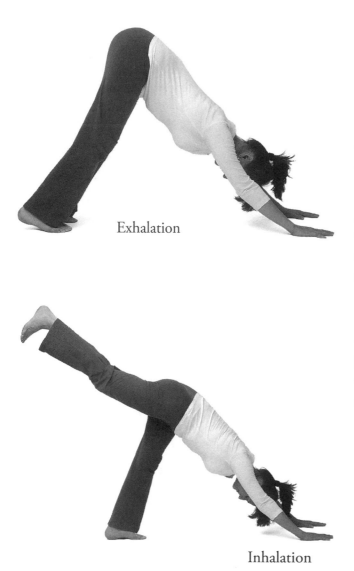

Exhalation

Inhalation

Effect
Strengthens the arm and shoulder muscles. Stretches the spine and lower back.

Instructions
Come on to all fours. The hands are placed slightly in front of the shoulder joints.

Exhaling
Move the buttocks upwards and raise the knees off the floor. Stretch both arms and bend the knees slightly.

Inhaling
Stretch the spine. Raise the right leg and stretch upwards with the heel, without tilting the pelvis to the side. Take care not to overstretch the arms or strain the shoulder and elbow joints (see unhealthy postures).

Repetition: 6 × each side

Note: If you have sensitive wrists this exercise may be too great a strain. In this case carry out the exercise with the support of the lower arms and carry the weight on the forearms.

8. Ardha Dhanurasana

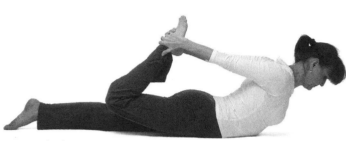

Inhalation

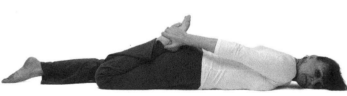

Exhalation

Effect
Stretches the chest and the front thigh and abdominal muscles. Strengthens the back extensor muscles and shoulder blade muscles. Has an energising effect.

Instructions
Lie on your front. Place the forehead on the floor and bend the right knee. Both hands are around the right ankle.

Inhaling
Raise the head and the chest. Pull the ankle gently with both hands to strengthen the shoulder blade muscles.

Exhaling
Come back into the starting position and turn the head alternately to the right and left.

Repetition: 8-10 × each side

Note: If you cannot hold the ankle, hold on to the back of your trousers with the fingers of the right hand.

9. Paschimottanasana

Effect
Stretches and balances the lower back and the shoulder blade muscles.

Instructions
Sit in an upright position and bend the knee.

Inhaling
Keep the pelvis straight. Activate the pelvic floor and stretch the spine. At the same time, raise the arms out to the sides up to shoulder height.

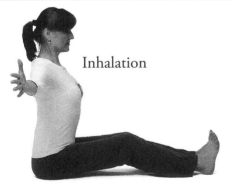

Inhalation

Exhaling
Bend forward slightly and place the stomach on the thigh. Bend the knee and place the hands on the floor to the sides, next to the legs.

Repetition: × 8-10

Note: To keep the pelvis straight you may need a cushion for support.

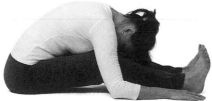

Exhalation

10. Catuspadapitham

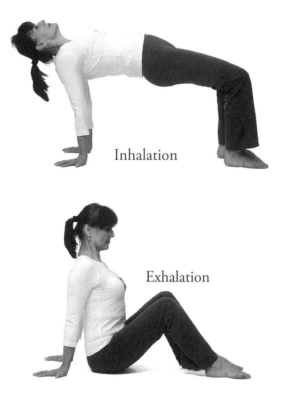

Inhalation

Exhalation

Effect
Strengthens the arm, shoulder and rhomboid muscles, as well as the neck and back extensor muscles. Opens the chest.

Instructions
Sit upright with feet flat on the floor. Place the hands on the floor next to the buttocks to support the body. The fingers and wrists are pointing outwards.

Inhaling
Raise the buttocks and stretch the arms. It is easier to open the chest if the fingers are pointing backwards away from the body.

Exhaling
Lower the buttocks on to the floor.

Repetition: × 8-10, then remain for 3 breaths

Note: If you have sensitive wrists, find a position for the hands that does not cause any pain. You may wish to use the fists for support. It is vital to keep the neck active and not let it fall backwards.

11. Variant of Ardha Matsyendrasana

Effect
Mobilises and strengthens the upper back, sternocleidomastoid and rhomboid muscles.

Instructions
Remain in an upright sitting position. The knee is bent and the right sole of the foot is touching the inside of the left thigh. The left leg is stretched out. The left hand is placed on the left shin and the right hand is behind, next to the buttock.

Exhaling
Turn the spine and right shoulder to the right. At the same time, turn the head to the left. The pelvis remains stable and is not rotated. With each inhalation, increase the straightening of the spine and the strengthening of the rhomboid muscles.

Repetition: Remain for 6-8 breaths

Note: For optimum straightening of the pelvis and spine, you may use a cushion to sit on. The spiralling counter-movement in the spine enables optimum opening of the chest and stretches the intercostal muscles.

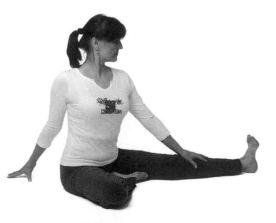

12. Siddhasana

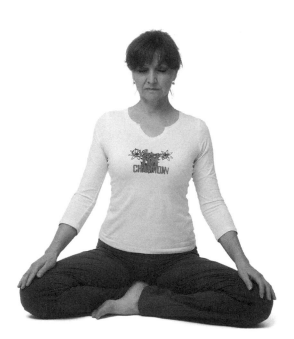

Effect
Builds up energy through extended inhalation and holding of the breath. Strengthens the respiratory muscles.

Instructions
Sit on a cushion. The right heel is close to the cushion. The left heel is placed in front of the right foot. Both legs are rotated outwards. Change the position of your legs in the sitting posture now and again, to avoid any muscular imbalances.

Breathing rhythm
Inhalation: 4 seconds, 2 second pause (fullness of the breath)
Inhalation: 4 seconds
Exhalation: 8 seconds
Repetition: × 6

Breathing rhythm
Inhalation: 6 seconds,2 second pause (fullness of the breath)\
Inhalation: 6 seconds
Exhalation: 12 seconds
Repetition: × 8

Breathing rhythm
Inhalation: 4 seconds 2 second pause (fullness of the breath)
Inhalation: 4 seconds
Exhalation: 8 seconds
Repetition: × 4 Also, watch the breath and the effect on your mind.

Note:
Only increase the inhalation if you feel all right. Respect how you feel at that moment and observe your limitations. If you have high blood pressure or a heart complaint, do not hold your breath. If you already have a large inhalation volume, you can increase the length of the inhalation.

Chapter 3: Yoga therapy for chronic conditions

There are no universally applicable yoga exercises or Ayurveda tips for chronic complaints and diseases. As the same conditions are manifested individually in each person, specific adaptation of the yoga practice and Ayurveda tips are important for a successful outcome. However, the yoga programme and Ayurveda recommendations presented here may achieve a very good result. They are simple, safe exercises you can try out for yourself. If you are unsure whether or not you can and should do these, please ask your doctor for advice.

Yoga programme for asthma
Effects

- Stretches the sides of the ribs and chest muscles.

- Stretches the small and large chest muscles.

- Relaxes the diaphragm.

- Lengthens the exhalation

- Mobilises the thoracic spine and ribs.

- Encourages trust and awareness of your own breathing rhythm

- Calms the nervous system and mind

1. Chakravakasana

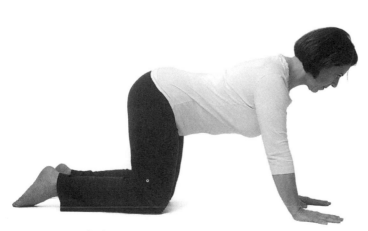

Inhalation

Effect
Stretches the lower back and mobilises the thoracic spine.

Instructions
Come on to all fours. The hips and knees are in alignment. Place the wrists a little in front of the shoulder joints.

Inhaling
Extend the spine and open the chest by slightly raising the breastbone.

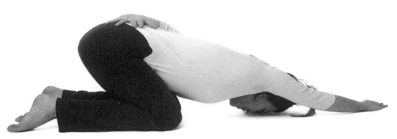

Exhaling

Round the lower back and move the buttocks towards the heels. At the same time, place the back of the left hand on the lower back and the forehead on the floor.

Repetition: 6 × each side

Exhalation

2. Vajrasana

Inhalation

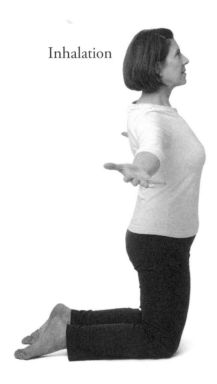

Effect

Stretches the sides of the shoulder and rib muscles. Stretches the small and large chest muscles.

Instructions

Come into a kneeling position. If the knees are sensitive to pressure in this position, place a blanket under the knees.

Inhaling

Raise both arms out to the sides to shoulder height. Open the hands and splay the fingers.

Exhaling

Come into a forward bend and turn the upper body to the left, placing the right palm on the floor. Place the back of the left hand on the sacrum. Bring the buttocks almost to the heels to strengthen the stretch in the upper back.

Repetition: 6 × each side and hold for 3 breaths

Exhalation

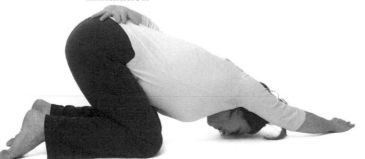

3. Vinyasa Tadasana and Ardha Utkatasana

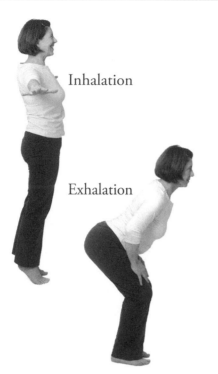

Inhalation

Exhalation

Effect
Extends the exhalation and relaxes the diaphragm.

Instructions
Come into an upright standing position with the feet hip width apart.

Inhaling
Lift the heels from the floor and raise both arms out to the sides to shoulder height.

Exhaling
Go into the half squat and bend the knees only so far that you can still see the toes and the front of the foot. Place the hands on the thigh. Hum "ha" at the same time.

Repetition: × 8

Note: Discover your own breathing rhythm and adapt the exercise to the breath. You can also take an interim breath.

4. Virabhdrasana and Parshva Uttanasana

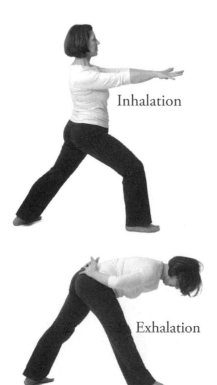

Inhalation

Exhalation

Effect
Stretches the ribs and shoulder blade muscles.

Instructions
In the upright standing position with the feet hip width apart, turn the left leg out, so that the left foot is pointing 45 degrees outwards. Now take a large step forwards with the right foot and bend the right leg.

Inhaling
Raise both arms in front of the body to shoulder height. Relax the shoulders downwards.

Exhaling
Come into a half forward bend and bring the back of the hand to the lower back. Round the upper back a little towards the end of the movement.

Repetition: 8 × each side

5. Variant of Utthita Trikonasana

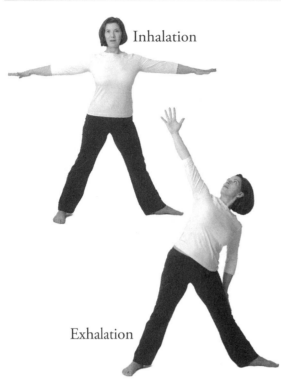

Inhalation

Exhalation

Effect

Stretches the flanks as well as the side rib muscles. Mobilises the ribs and chest.

Instructions

In the upright standing position, turn the right thigh out, so that the right foot is pointing 90 degrees outwards, and take a large step backwards with the foot. The pelvis is directed out to the side.

Inhaling

Raise both arms out to the sides up to shoulder height.

Exhaling

Bring the upper body down to the left side. Place the left hand on the thigh. Stretch the right arm upwards to the side and at the same time turn the spine and the head in the direction of the right hand.

Repetition: 8 × each side

6. Variant of Virabhadrasana

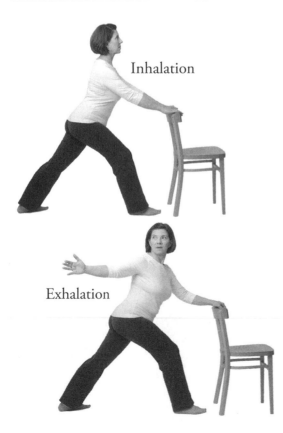

Inhalation

Exhalation

Effect

Mobilises the thoracic spine and the ribs.

Instructions

Take a chair for this exercise and hold on to the back of the chair with both hands. Turn the left leg 45 degrees outwards and take a step backwards with the left foot.

Inhaling

Bend the right knee and raise the breastbone to stretch the thoracic spine. Rest both hands on the back of the chair.

Exhaling

Move the right arm right and backwards and turn the upper body to the right. The pelvis remains stable and the rotation is from the thoracic spine.

Repetition: 8 × each side

7. Chakravakasana

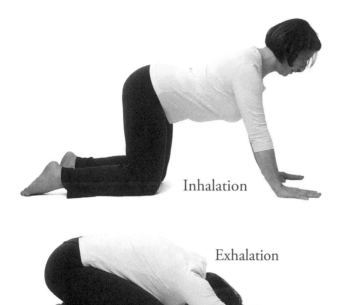

Inhalation

Exhalation

Effect
Lengthens the exhalation and relaxes the mind.

Instructions
Come on to all fours. Knees and hips are in alignment. The wrists are placed a little in front of the shoulder joints.

Inhaling
Lengthen the spine and open the chest by raising the breastbone a little.

Exhaling
Round the lower back and lower the buttocks towards the heels whilst softly humming an "ooh" sound.

Repetition: × 8-10

8. Variant of Ardha Matsyendrasana

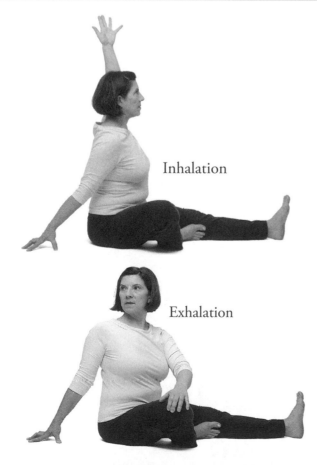

Inhalation

Exhalation

Effect
Stretches the spine and mobilises the thoracic spine.

Instructions
Sit in an upright position and move the right knee outwards to the right. The left leg is stretched out to the front. You may sit on a cushion for optimum straightening of the spine.

Inhaling
Raise the left arm and stretch it above the head.

Exhaling
Turn the chest on the right side and put the left hand on the right knee, while placing the fingertips of the right hand on the floor to the right.

Repetition: 6 × each side and remain in the rotation for 3 breaths.

Note: The pelvis remains stable and the twist comes from the thoracic spine

9. Paschimottanasana

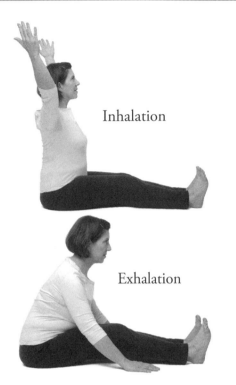

Inhalation

Exhalation

Effect
Balances and stretches the lower back.

Instructions
Stretch both legs out forwards in the upright sitting position.

Inhaling
Stretch both arms above the head.

Exhaling
Come into a gentle forward bend with bent knees.

Repetition: × 8

10. Sitting position on a chair

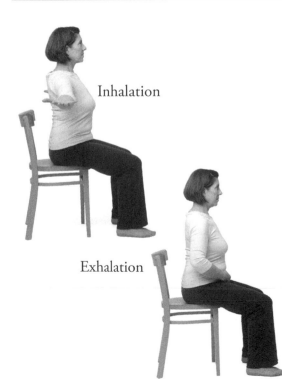

Inhalation

Exhalation

Effect
Deepens abdominal breathing and lengthens the exhalation. Relaxes the diaphragm and calms the mind.

Instructions
Sit on a chair for optimum alignment of the spine.

Inhaling
Raise the arms out to the sides and breathe in gently.

Exhaling
Lower the arms and place the hands on the abdomen. Breathe out slowly and with awareness and discover your own breathing rhythm. Increase the exhalation very subtly without straining.

Repetition: × 10

11. Same position

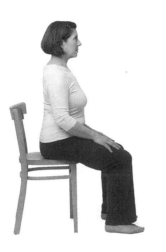

Effect
Calms the mind and deepens the exhalation.

Instructions
Place the hands on the thighs.

Inhaling
Breathe quite freely without straining.

Exhaling
Gently sound "om".

Ayurveda recommendations for asthma

Asthma results in impaired breathing, an increase in the number of breaths and rattling, whistling noises are produced when breathing. The bronchial tubes narrow and sometimes are inflamed, excreting secretions. If the mucus cannot be coughed up, the bronchi contract, which can lead to shortness of breath or even suffocation.

Ayurveda equates bronchial asthma with *kapha* disruption. The *kapha dosha* falls out of balance AND the body begins to form too much mucus, which often remains deposited in the bronchi. Ayurveda medicine therefore seeks to inhibit the formation of mucus and thus free the body of an excess of it.

Ayurveda traces problems with the airways back to the following causes irregular eating, undigested food, dry food, cold water, dust, smoke, excessive travel and living in extremely cold countries.

Asthma worsens with the change of seasons and weather and attacks usually occur at night. Patients suffer from shortness of breath when lying down, which improves when sitting up. If asthma remains untreated,

complications may arise on top of difficulties in inhaling and managing everyday tasks, such as hoarseness, coughing, cardiac asthma and tuberculosis.

Internal medicine and suggested remedies

A mix of three herbs – *triphala* – to stimulate expulsion from the intestine take 3 teaspoons once a day with some tea or hot water. This remedy is suitable for the long-term prevention of asthma

Twice a day, put 1 teaspoon of cinnamon and ¼ teaspoon of *trikatu* (black pepper, long pepper and ginger in equal parts) in a cup with boiling water and let it draw for 10 minutes. Add 1 teaspoon of honey before drinking.

For detoxification we recommend taking 4 capsules of *guggulu* (Indian tree gum) three × a day with some Vata tea or fresh nettle mixed with berries, water, ginger and cinnamon, with up to 1 litre of water, to be chewed daily by the spoonful. In the same way, fresh ribwort can be taken to counter bronchial illnesses. This is mixed with berries, water, ginger and cinnamon, with up to 1 litre of water a day, chewed daily by the spoonful.

Diet and lifestyle

Asthmatics should avoid the following

- Meals at night-time

- All milk products except butter and ghee

- Foods with a sour taste

- Foods with carbohydrates containing glutens (wheat, rye, spelt, barley and oats)

- Dry foods and baked goods

- Bananas and guava

- Sweet foods containing sugar

- Cold food and cold drinks

- Cold weather and travel in general

- Hot, bitter flavours are better, e.g. ginger tea, miso soup and chilli bean dishes.

During the asthma attack, small amounts of food should be consumed that are hot, light and fluid. Meals should be appetising and easy to digest (ginger is very useful here) and should be eaten in the early evening. Warm water should be drunk and should also be the choice for baths and showers.

Yoga

The yoga exercises will bring calm and should therefore be practised regularly. They will relax the diaphragm and respiratory muscles and should therefore be carried out in a way that they will not trigger any problems. Asthmatics should avoid intensive breathing exercises.

Yoga practice for high blood pressure

Effects

- Releases neck tension.

- Stretches the shoulder muscles.

- Mobilises and stretches the thoracic spine.

- Extends the exhalation and calms the nervous system.

- Relaxes the muscles in the entire body.

- Creates space for awareness of the breath

- Encourages relaxation and mental clarity.

1. Sukhasana

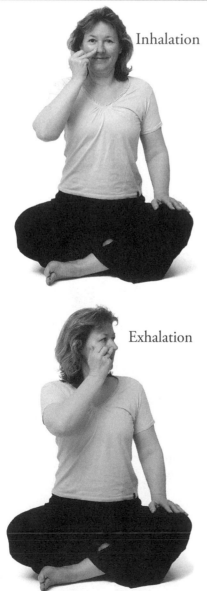

Inhalation

Exhalation

Effect
Balancing Effect on the body and mind. Releases neck tension.

Instructions
Sit on a cushion. The right heel is close to the cushion. The left is placed forward. Both feet are pointing outwards. Close the right nostril with the right ring finger.

Inhaling
Inhale slowly through the open left nostril.

Exhaling
Turn the head to the left and exhale through the left nostril at the same time.

Repetition: × 8. Then change the leg position, ring finger and rotation and repeat 8 × the other side.

2. Chakravakasana

Inhalation

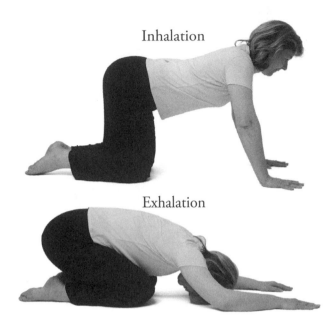

Exhalation

Effect
Stretches the lower back and lengthens the exhalation through sound.

Instructions
Come on to all fours. The hips and knees are in alignment. The hands are placed slightly in front of the shoulder joints.

Inhaling
Extend the spine and open the chest.

Exhaling
Begin to round the lower back and sound a deep "ooh", as the buttocks sink back to the heels.

Repetition: × 12

3. Eka Pada Ustrasana

Inhalation

Exhalation

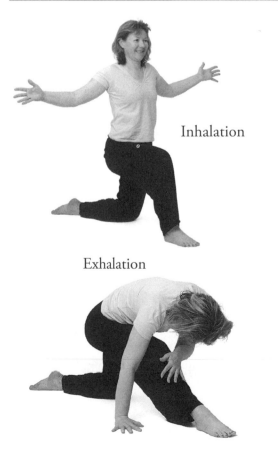

Effect
Stretches the chest, shoulder blades and lower back muscles.

Instructions
Come into a kneeling position and step the right foot forward on the floor. The ankle and knee are in alignment.

Inhaling
Raise both arms out to the sides up to around the shoulder joints. The palms are facing forwards.

Exhaling
Come into the forward bend and place the left hand on the right shin. Position the right hand on the floor to give stability to the pose.

Repetition: 8 × each side

4. Vinyasa Tadasana and Ardha Utkatasana

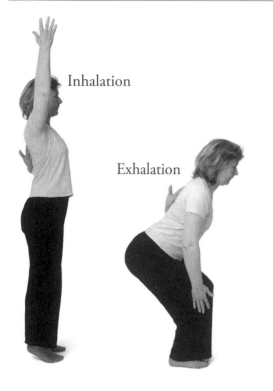

Inhalation

Exhalation

Effect
Stretches the spine. Stretches the outer shoulder blade and upper arm muscles,

Instructions
Come into the upright standing position with the feet hip width apart. Place the back of the left hand on the right shoulder blade.

Inhaling
Raise both heels from the floor and stretch the right arm to the side above the head.

Exhaling
Lower the heels and come into a semi-squat squat. Lower the right arm and place the right hand on the outside of the right knee.

Repetition: 8 × each side

5. Variant of Vinyasa Virabhadrasana and Utthita Trikonasana

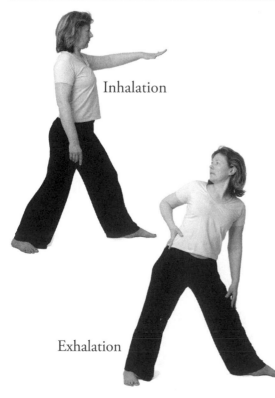

Inhalation

Exhalation

Effect
Mobilises the thoracic spine. Stretches the sides and rib muscles.

Instructions
From the upright standing position, turn the right leg out so that the right foot is pointing 45 degrees outwards. Now take a big step forward with the left foot and bend the left leg.

Inhaling
Raise the left arm to the front up to shoulder height.

Exhaling
Bend forward and turn the upper body to the right. Place the left hand on the left thigh. Turn the head to the right. Place the right hand on the right side of the waist.

Repetition: 6 × each side and remain in the turn for three breaths

6. Ardha Parshva Uttanasana

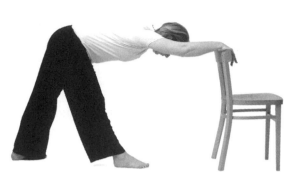

Effect
Stretches the back muscles and extends the spine. Deepens the exhalation and calms the mind.

Instructions
From the upright standing position, turn the left leg out so that the left foot is pointing 45 degrees outwards. Now take a large step forwards with the right foot. Take a chair and Exhaling, bend forwards. Support yourself by placing both hands on the back of the chair. Stretch the spine and consciously deepen the slow exhalation.

Repetition: Remain in the posture for 6 breaths on each side.

7. Samasthiti

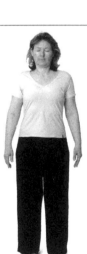

Effect
Awareness of the breath and calming of the mind.

Instructions
Come back into the symmetrical standing position with the feet hip width apart. Find the upright position and watch your breath.

Repetition: Remain in this position for about a minute.

8. Variant of Ardha Matsyendrasana

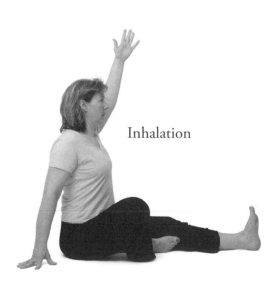

Inhalation

Effect
Mobilises the thoracic spine and neck. Strengthens the upper back. Releases neck tension.

Instructions
Sit in an upright position, stretch the left leg forward and bend the right leg, so that the right knee is pointing outwards. For optimum straightening of the spine you may sit on a cushion.

Inhaling
Stretch the left arm above the head and straighten the spine.

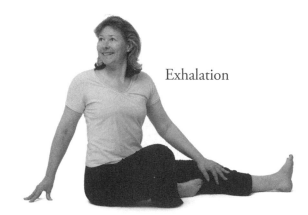

Exhalation

Exhaling

Turn the spine and head to the right. Place the left hand on the left knee. The fingertips of the right hand are on the floor on the right side. The pelvis remains stable. The turning movement is in the upper back only.

Repetition: 6 × each side and remain in the rotation for 3 breaths

Note: Ensure that you keep the spine straight for the rotation. The pelvis remains stable and the shoulder blades relaxed.

9. Urdhva Prasarita Padasana

Inhalation

Exhalation

Effect

Balances and stretches the lower back. Extends the exhalation through sounding.

Instructions

Lie on your back and place the feet on the floor. Place the arms next to the body.

Inhaling

Raise both arms vertically and at the same time stretch the right leg upwards.

Exhaling

Sound out "om" and at the same time draw the knee towards the chest using both hands.

Repetition: 8 × each side

10. Shavasana

Effect

Extended exhalation and relaxation of the nervous system. Releases muscle tension and deep emotions.

Instructions

Lying on your back, place the arms next to the body. Exhale very slowly and with awareness. Relax the muscles from the back of the head to the heels. You may also wish to cover your eyes.

Repetition: Remain in the position for 3-4 minutes.

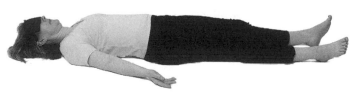

Ayurveda recommendations for high blood pressure (hypertension)

Blood flows ideally at a pressure of around 120/80 mmHg through the veins and arteries. If the blood pressure is above 140/90 mmHg a doctor should be consulted and medicine taken to control the blood pressure. Hypertension, if it continues over a long period, has a negative effect on the kidneys, brain, heart, eyes and nervous system and causes heart disease. Ayurveda regards high blood pressure in most cases as the result of an over-acidified body, a clogged digestive tract, clotted vessels and an over-production of stress hormones. Hypertension may affect any type of constitution. However, it is manifested in different ways, i.e. in the *vata dosha* it rises and falls suddenly, in the *pitta dosha* it arises as a complication from a liver dysfunction and in the *kapha dosha* it displays itself constantly and in association with obesity and tiredness.

Internal medicine and suggested remedies

Rauwolfia serpentina is suitable as an alternative to blood-pressure reducing aids. One capsule is to be taken twice a day.

To regulate high blood pressure, you can eat a piece of water melon with a pinch of cardamom and a pinch of coriander. This has a slightly diuretic effect. Alternatively, mix 1 teaspoon of coriander and a pinch of cardamom with a cup of freshly pressed peach juice. Drink this mixture two to three times a day. To improve the micro-circulation and free up the agglutination of blood cells, mix and purée fresh nettles with fruits and eat them thoroughly chewed up.

Diet and lifestyle

It is important to reduce your weight and clean your digestive tract. To reduce the craving for carbohydrates and sweet foods, consume a diet based on raw foods, which supplies the body with sufficient nutrition, organic minerals, enzymes and biophotons and which must therefore come from high-quality, organically-grown foods. The enteric vessels will then be freed up and gluten-containing carbohydrates and animal proteins, which form acid, should be largely avoided.

- People with high blood pressure should therefore give up the following foods

- Wheat, rye, spelt, barley, oats, potatoes, sweet potatoes, peanuts, sago and all fried food, meat, eggs, cheese, butter, bananas, figs, mangoes, jack fruit and cherimoya.

- People with high blood pressure should ideally eat the following

- Limes, oranges, water melons, pomegranate, apples, Jambolana plums, amaranth, spinach, cabbage, cucumber, carrots, red beet, radishes, gooseberries, corn, chickpeas, cardamom, ginger, black pepper, black mustard seeds, turmeric and cumin.

- Vital foods should not be heated up so that they retain their healthy ingredients. Adding wild herbs increases the density of these vital substances.

Yoga, meditation and exercise

Yoga and meditation should be carried out in a calming and relaxing way and practised daily. Heavy yoga practice and certain yoga postures may worsen the complaint. Besides this, it is important to move around for 30 to 60 minutes every day to reduce the body weight and control the high blood pressure.

Yoga programme to stimulate digestion and encourage emotional stability

Effects

- Relaxes the abdominal muscles.

- Strengthens the diagonal, straight and deep-seated abdominal muscles

- Strengthens the buttock and back extensor muscles.

- Strengthens the fronts, backs and sides of the thigh muscles.

- Straightens the spine.

- Stimulates suppressed feelings. Intensifies the digestion process (agni) via "ra" sounds and breathing techniques.

- Encourages emotional stability and inner strength

1. Urdhva Prasarita Padasana

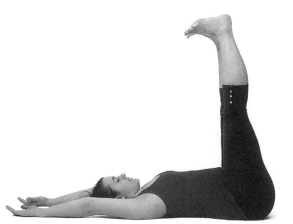

Inhalation

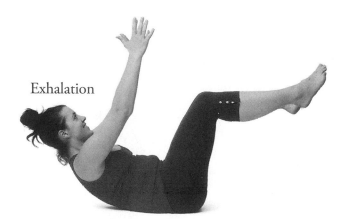

Exhalation

Effect
Strengthens the straight abdominal muscles and stretches the spine

Instructions
Lie on your back with the feet hip width apart.

Inhaling
Stretch both arms above the head and stretch both legs up vertically at the same time.

Exhaling
Roll the upper body slowly up from the floor and stretch both arms upwards vertically. At the same time, bend both legs. The heels and knees are in alignment.

Repetition: × 10-12

Note: If you have neck problems, you can place both hands at the back of the head when coming up, to reduce the strain on the neck.

2. Variant of Chakravakasana

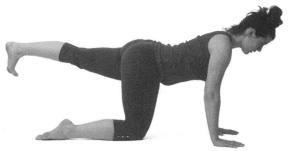

Inhalation

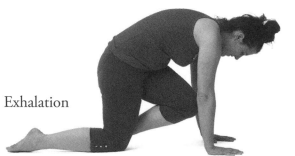

Exhalation

Effect
Strengthens the buttocks, back extensor muscles and diagonal abdominal muscles

Instructions
Come on to all fours. hips and knees are in alignment. Place the wrists a little in front of the shoulder joints.

Inhaling
Stretch the left leg backwards and flexthe foot. Emphasise the extension of the spine and avoid too much curvature (hollowing) of the lumbar spine.

Exhaling
Bend the left leg and move the left knee towards the right elbow. Round the spine at the same time.

Repetition: 8 × each side

3. Anantasana

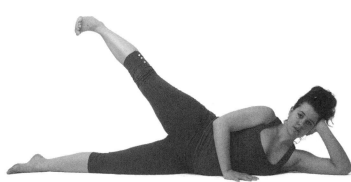

Inhalation

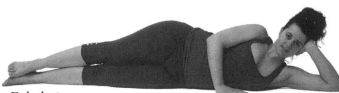

Exhalation

Effect
Strengthens the sides of the thighs and buttock muscles.

Instructions
Lie on your side with the left side of your body in contact with the floor. The shoulder, pelvis and outstretched legs are in alignment. Support the head with the left hand.

Inhaling
Raise the right leg to the side about a metre high and turn the right foot inwards.

Exhaling
Lower the right leg and place it on the left leg.

Repetition: 8 × each side

4. Vinyasa Tadasana and Ardha Utkatasana

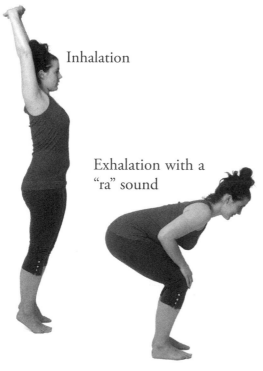

Inhalation

Exhalation with a "ra" sound

Effect
Strengthens the thigh and buttock muscles. Stimulates the digestive system (agni).

Instructions
Place the feet hip width apart.

Inhaling
Raise the heels off the floor and stretch both arms in front of the body and above the head. The fingers are interlocked and the palms are facing upwards.

Exhaling
Lower the heels and bend both legs to come into a semi-squat. Place the palms on the thighs. Sound "ra" with a strong voice. Do not move the knee too far forwards and press the heels firmly into the floor.

Repetition: × 10

5. Variant of Parshva Konasana

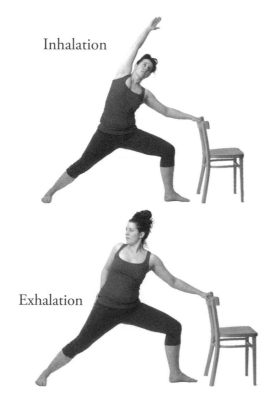

Inhalation

Exhalation

Effect
Stretches the sides of the abdomen and the trunk muscles.

Instructions
Come into a standing position with the legs splayed wide apart. The left foot is turned 90 degrees outwards. The left leg is bent. Come into a sideways bend and support the left hand on the back of a chair.

Inhaling
Move the right arm to the side above the head and stretch the right side of the body.

Exhaling
Lower the right arm and place the hand on the waist. At the same time turn the head and the chest to the right.

Repetition: 8 × each side

6. Variant of Utthita Eka Padangusthasana

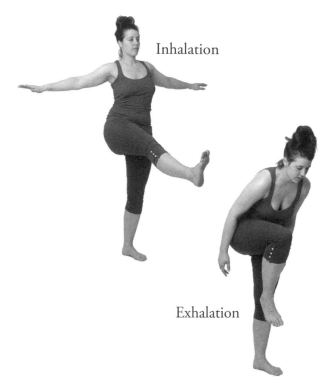

Inhalation

Exhalation

Effect
Strengthens the thigh and side buttock muscles.

Instructions
Come into an upright standing position with the feet hip width apart.

Inhaling
Raise both arms out to the sides to shoulder height and stretch the right leg forward horizontally. The spine remains as straight as possible.

Exhaling
Lower the arms and bend the right leg. Move the right knee towards the abdomen and round the upper body.

Repetition: 8 × each side

Note: You may rest both hands on the back of a chair to reduce the strain on the knee and gain more stability.

7. Variant of Natarajasana

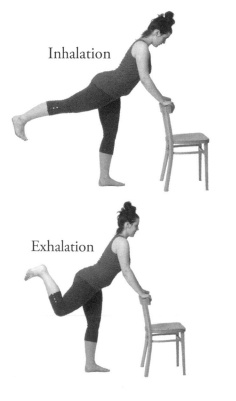

Inhalation

Exhalation

Effect
Strengthens the backs of the thighs, the buttocks and back extensor muscles

Instructions
Remain in the upright standing position with the feet hip width apart and rest both hands on the back of a chair.

Inhaling
Come into a gentle forward bend and stretch the right leg backwards. Lengthen the lower back and avoid making too much of a hollow by not raising the right leg too far.

Exhaling
Bend the right leg and bring the right heel towards the buttock.

Repetition: 8 × each side

8. Tadasana with active breath

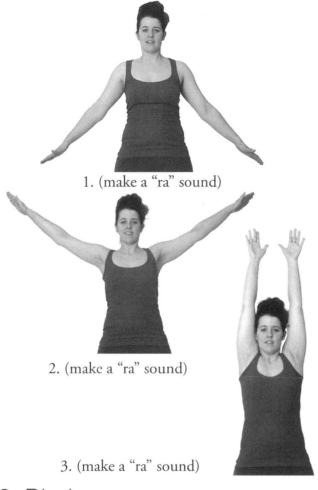

1. (make a "ra" sound)

2. (make a "ra" sound)

3. (make a "ra" sound)

Effect
Stimulates the digestive system and releases suppressed feelings.

Instructions
Remain in the upright standing position with the feet hip width apart.

Inhaling
Raise both arms to the sides and slightly upwards quickly with a strong "ra" sound. Then bring the arms slightly higher with a "ra" sound and to finish, stretch both arms above the head with a strong "ra".

Exhaling
Lower the arms to the sides and exhale very slowly.

Repetition: 6 ×

Note: If you have high blood pressure and suffer from migraines, do the exercise gently, by coming up in two steps and sounding the "ra" softly.

9. Bhujangasana

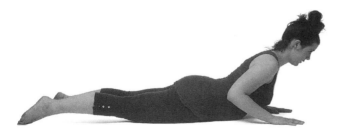

Effect
Strengthens the lower back and stimulates the digestion.

Instructions
Lie on your front. The hands are placed by the shoulders. Turn the head to the right.

Inhaling
Raise the upper body and open the chest. Do not put any pressure on the hands but rise up using the strength of the lower back.

Repetition: Remain in the position for 4-6 breaths.

Note: Ensure that you keep the neck long in this position and pay attention to the opening of the chest.

10. Vinyasa Urdhva Prasarita Padasana and Jathara Parivritti

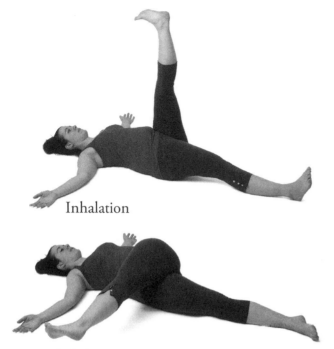

Inhalation

Exhalation

Effect
Strengthens the sides of the abdomen and the buttock muscles. Strengthens the lower back.

Instructions
Lie on your back with outstretched legs. Stretch the arms out to the sides from the body.

Inhaling
Stretch the left leg upwards vertically.

Exhaling
Move the stretched left leg to the right without placing the foot completely on the floor. Now,

Inhaling, come back on to the starting position.

Repetition: 8 × each side

Note: If you have back pain, bend the leg Exhaling and move the knee just slightly to the side. Avoid strong rotations in the lower back.

11. Paschimottanasana

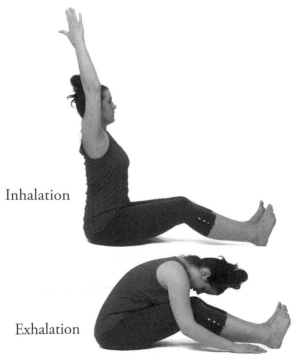

Inhalation

Exhalation

Effect
Gently stretches the lower back and is a balancing posture.

Instructions
Come into the sitting position with legs stretched forward.

Inhaling
Stretch both arms above the head and straighten the spine.

Exhaling
Come into a gentle forward bend with bent knees.

Repetition: × 10

12. Siddhasana with Kabalabhati

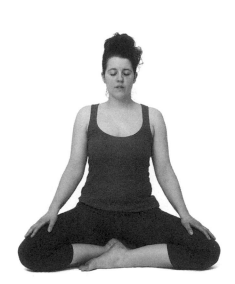

Effect
Stimulates the digestion and releases suppressed feelings. Purging and detoxifying.

Instructions
Sit on a cushion. Move the right knee outwards and place the right heel close to the cushion. Move the left knee outwards and place the left heel in front of the right heel. Exhaling, pull the abdominal wall inwards quickly. Inhale passively through the nose.

Repetition
Breathe quickly 18 times, then take 3 deep breaths. 3-4 rounds

Note: Do not do Kabalabhati if you have a serious heart condition or high blood pressure. If you feel a tendency to faint, do the exercise carefully.

13. Siddhasana

Effect
Focuses the mind. Encourages emotional stability and inner strength.

Instructions
From the same sitting position, place the left palm on the navel. Place the right palm on the left one. Close your eyes and focus your attention under the left hand in the abdominal area. Be aware of your sensitivities, thoughts and feelings, pay attention to them and simply let them be.

Repetition: 3-5 minutes

Ayurveda recommendations for overweight and obesity

Obesity is a chronic disease whereby the fatty tissue in the body increases and is retained. Obesity is caused by excessive consumption of foods that are high in calories, particularly foods that are sweet, fatty, cold and with high meat content, as well as by lack of exercise or physical work, excessive daily breaks, genetic disorders and/or hormonal imbalances in men and women. People who suffer from obesity have difficulties carrying out their daily work. They usually sweat excessively, their abdominal area is above average in size, they suffer from breathlessness at the least exertion, are phlegmatic and have difficulties being sexually active. They usually suffer from excessive sensations of thirst and constant hunger. If obesity is not treated it can led to diabetes, heart problems, high blood pressure, arthrosis and strokes. Ayurveda distinguishes between seven tissues (*dhatus*). With obesity only meda, the fat tissue is built up, while bone tissue, nerves and reproductive tissues are not nourished. Overweight, which is due to a slow metabolism, is viewed as an illness of the *kapha dosha*

Internal medicine and suggested remedies

To stimulate the digestive system, cut 1 piece of fresh ginger, drizzle a few drops of lime and a pinch of salt on it and chew it slowly. Take this before every meal.

As a substitute for high-calorie meals and to reduce the body weight, the following fresh food is recommended, puréed in a food-mixer

Two-thirds (of the content of the mix) is green leaf salad, (e.g. spinach leaves, green cabbage, parsley, rocket or mangold, grown organically) or wild herb leaves (ground elder, dandelion, white chenopod, ribwort, ground ivy, cabbage thistle and particularly nettles),- 2 tablespoons of primal essence microminerals,- Fruits (e.g. 1 cup of frozen or fresh raspberries, 2 to 6 dates, juice of a lemon, 1 ripe banana or 1 orange),- 1 piece of fresh ginger, 1 tablespoon of cinnamon, ½ teaspoon of cardamom,- Half fill the container with water and purée.- Add sunflower seeds or coconut flakes as required.

Diet and lifestyle

Diet is also a decisive factor to control body weight and counter different diseases. This is more to do with the quality of the food rather than the quantity.

People who are overweight should avoid the following foods

- Sweets and sweet foods of all kinds, dairy products except butter and cream, wheat, rye, spelt, oats, barley, potatoes, sweet potatoes, peanuts, sago, all fried foods, meat, eggs, cheese, butter, bananas, figs, mangoes, jack fruits and cherimoya.

- People who are overweight should ideally consume the following foods

- All vegetables that can be eaten raw, amaranth, spinach, cabbage, cucumbers, carrots, red beet, radishes, gooseberries, corn, chickpeas, cardamom, ginger, pepper, black mustard seeds, turmeric and cumin. Lukewarm or hot water should be drunk constantly. Hot water with honey is also recommended for the mornings.

Yoga and exercise

The yoga exercises should be adapted to the individual mobility or carried out with the guidance of a qualified yoga teacher. It is also necessary to exercise for 30 to 60 minutes every day to reduce the body weight.

Yoga programme for reducing stress
Effect

- Extended exhalation

- Calms the nervous system

- Relieves back tension

- Concentrates and focuses the mind

- Reduces the influx of thoughts

- Brings a connection with inner peace and calm

1. Shavasana

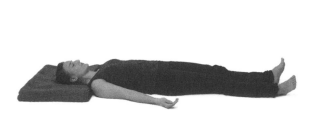

Effect
Relaxes and extends the exhalation.

Instructions
Lie on your back. Place the arms at the sides next to the body. Place a blanket under the back of the head and neck.

Inhaling
Take a very relaxed breath in.

Exhaling
Consciously extend the exhalation without straining.

Repetition: 2-3 minutes

Note: If it feels more comfortable for the neck, you may place a blanket under the back of the head. If you have tension or pain in the lower back, place the feet on the floor and move them close to the buttocks.

2. Urdhva Prasarita Padasana

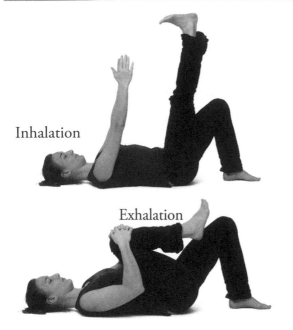

Inhalation

Exhalation

Effect
Stretches and relaxes the lower back.

Instructions
Lying on your back, place the feet on the floor hip width apart. The arms are at the sides next to the body.

Inhaling
Raise both arms and stretch the right leg vertically upwards.

Exhaling
Bend the right leg and pull the right knee towards the chest using both hands.

Repetition: 8 × each side

3. Posture Chakravakasana

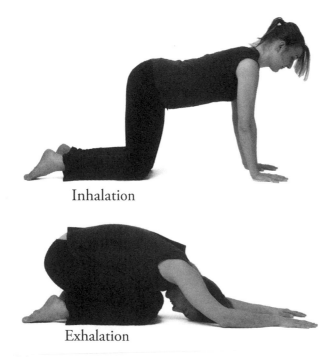

Inhalation

Exhalation

Effect
Extended exhalation and calms of the mind by emptying the breath

Instructions
Come on to all fours. The hips and knees are in alignment. Place the hands a little in front of the shoulder joints.

Inhaling
Lengthen the spine and raise the breastbone to open the chest.

Exhaling
Exhale slowly with awareness and then take a few seconds before inhaling.

Repetition: 8 × and remain in the second position for 3 breaths

Note: If you suffer from any health problems such as asthma, high blood pressure or heart complaints, it is not a good idea to hold the breath.

4. Eka Pada Ustrasana

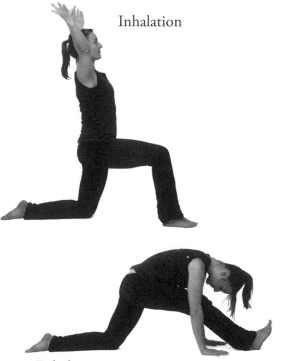

Inhalation

Exhalation.
At the end, remail for 3 breaths

Effect
Stretches the front and back thigh muscles. Releases muscular tension in the buttocks and the lower back.

Instructions
From the kneeling position, step the right foot forwards. The ankle and knee are in alignment.

Inhaling
Raise and stretch both arms above the head and lengthen the spine.

Exhaling
Come into the forward bend and stretch the right leg as far as possible. Place the hands on the floor to give you support at the sides and stabilise the posture.

Repetition: 6 × each side and remain in the second position for 3 breaths.

Note: If the leg muscles are shortened, bend the front leg a little to optimise the forward bend.

5. Variant of Janu Shirshasana

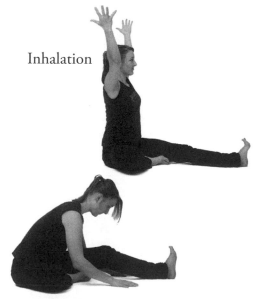

Inhalation

Exhalation.
At the end, remail for 4 breaths

Effect
Concentrates and focuses the mind.

Instructions
Come into an upright sitting position and move the right knee outwards. For optimum alignment of the spine and an Effective forward bend, you may wish to sit on a cushion.

Inhaling
Raise and stretch both arms above the head.

Exhaling
Come into a forward bend and sound a gentle "om". Bend the left knee.

Repetition: 8 × each side and remain for 4 breaths

6. Shavasana and Pranayama

Effect
Deepens the exhalation. Calms the nervous system and relaxes the mind.

Instructions
Lie on your back and place the arms at the sides next to the body. You may place a blanket under the head so that the neck remains long and relaxed.

A. Inhaling
The inhalation is always free and not forced in any way.

Exhaling
6 seconds, 6 times 8 seconds, 6 times 10 seconds, 6 times 12 seconds, 6 times 6 seconds, × 6

Note:
If the extension of the exhalation is too long for you, respect your limits and do not force the breath in any way.

Effect
Reduces stress and connects you with your inner peace. Reduces the influxof thoughts and focuses on what is important

B. Inhaling
Take very subtle and conscious breaths in.

Exhaling
Recite "om" in your mind. If thoughts distract you, come back to reciting "om" and be patient.

Repetition: 2-3 minutes. Then consciously take note of the effect it is having on your mind.

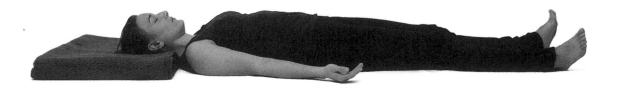

Ayurveda recommendations for stress

The mind plays an important part in stress-related complaints, as it coordinates the cooperation between the brain and the five senses of taste, smell, sight, touch and hearing.

Ayurveda explains stress as a *vata* disorder, which makes itself felt through problems such as head, joint and back pain, sleep disturbances, mood swings, flatulence, bloating and constipation. Professional and private pressure, shift work, lack of sleep, worry, over-activity, lack of or too much exercise, lack of rest and relaxation and dietary deficiencies bring the *vata dosha* out of balance, and therefore affect our physical and mental agility. The stress hormones cortisone, adrenaline and insulin are produced at higher than normal levels and overheat the body, which manifests as a permanent warning signal towards fight or flight. Over the long term, this excessive release of stress hormones may lead to a condition of burnout and depression. Short-term self-therapy via the sweet, salty, fatty and acidic foods, contained in fast food, sweets, fatty meat dishes, coffee, cake, fatty dairy products and spicy snacks, may balance out the *vata dosha* and thus the mental and physical processes of movement. However, in the medium term they lead to *kapha* disorders, so that lasting Ayurveda therapies are preferable.

Internal medicine and remedies

To reduce stress, prepare a tea with equal parts of camomile, comfrey and angelica and put this in a cup with boiled water. The tea has a calming effect. The daily ingestion of 2-3 tablespoons of wild herbs helps achieve inner relaxation and the reduction of stress hormones. These also give fresh energy and increase the resistance to stress.

Diet and lifestyle

It is important to undergo and maintain a daily routine from early morning up to going to bed, which is in accordance with the seasons. Hobbies such as painting, gardening, singing, writing books or writing poetry, have a grounding effect, as does connecting with people in groups, such as meeting friends or relatives, or attending clubs. Bad habits such as fast food should be replaced in favour of regular, high-quality meals. Diet, sleep and sex are the three pillars of life in their balanced form.

Yoga

Regular, calm yoga practice helps to deepen the connection to the inner self. Breathing and relaxation techniques have a short-term and long-term effect for stress-related complaints. The deep level of rest during meditation supports the reduction of stress knots and stress hormones.

Chapter 4: Healing and transformation

Self-acceptance

Every person encounters suffering in its many forms during their life, be it physical pain, illness, loss or painful experiences, such as disappointments and injuries. During such suffering we experience our restless, disparate mind, which constantly seeks diversion. This mental unrest takes up a lot of our energy and creates unfavourable preconditions for clear action. It also clouds our perception.

Patanjali, the creator of the yoga sutras, gives five causes (*kleshas* = mental barriers), which evince the different forms of suffering.

False understanding (*avidya*) is at the roots of misunderstanding and disappointments in life. It is only the "removal of the illusion" whereby we take away the veil of our perception and look reality in the face, which shows us this barrier clearly. Our wishes and ideals blithely lead us into not perceiving things clearly. Thus, every disappointment, even if painful, is also an opportunity to wake up. It shows us reality.

Ego-attachment (*asmita*) leads to a false perception of who and what we really are. Instead of perceiving our true "self", we cling to our body and identify with our mind. Ego-thinking leads us to believe that we are right. Arrogance, egotism, vanity, lack of humour and self-pity are typical signs of strong ego-attachment.

Greed (*raga*) signifies the desire to satisfy our needs through things and recognition. We can see in life every day how longing influences human reactions and actions. Wishing and envy produce expectations within us by which we direct our actions in order to fulfil these.

Aversion and avoidance (*dvesa*) are elements we meet constantly in life. Often we are not ready to accept the moment as it is. We judge experiences as unpleasant and try to avoid them although they are part of life. Strong aversion may lead to hate, which makes us blind. We can see what hate-filled people are capable of, for example, in wars, which cost the lives of many.

Fear (*abhinivesa*) is a feeling that we encounter again and again in many life situations. With illnesses and in our work and relationships, worries can weaken our life energy. We often repress them or are unsure how to circumvent them. The many ways in which we can meet our fears require honesty and the courage for us to show our vulnerability. It is certainly no coincidence that it is generally more difficult for men than for women to speak openly about their worries and show their weaknesses.

If we are prepared to accept that suffering exists, we are creating a good basis to see it and accept it in ourselves. Accepting suffering is the first step on the path towards healing and transformation. This self-acceptance helps us to alleviate suffering because we are no longer fighting against it.

This opens up the way to healing characteristics such as compassion, tranquillity, humility and modesty. Yoga is a path towards not identifying with suffering. Recently, severe toothache helped me to practise the "yoga truth" of self-acceptance beautifully. Instead of fighting against the pain, I enjoyed peacefulness and experienced my vulnerability. Accepting our putative weaknesses is a good exercise for deploying self-acceptance at a practical level. We free ourselves from donning masks and no longer live with the constant anxiety of being exposed – a game of hide-and-seek that saps our energy and reduces our enjoyment of life. Through the self-acceptance we experience, we can recognise the extent to which we are at peace. It also liberates us from the worry of not being loved and gives us the facility to live authentically. Its positive side-effect is that it reduces our complaining, annoyance and need to be in the right.

When we are attentive, it is possible for us to recognise when our thoughts are moving towards non-acceptance. With mental clarity we can decide how we can circumvent such thoughts. This freedom of conscious choice gives us wings to be able to master the most difficult situation calmly. You must therefore accept your body and your personality. It is worth it at all events. Each new day brings you countless situations to exercise acceptance. Use the opportunities!

Self-reflection

The second step towards healing and transformation is loving reflection. Viewing life with an open mind and without categorising is the true art of living. I will now outline a self-reflection exercise. Please read the text first, before doing the exercise. Place both hands on your abdominal wall. Become aware of the movement of the abdominal wall. If you are diverted by thoughts coming into your mind, simply direct your attention back to your abdomen. Remain in this exercise for a minute. Be accepting if your thoughts stray.

Now become aware of the feeling in your body. Sense which area of the body requires your attention. Direct your awareness to this area and inhale and exhale there consciously. Keep doing this exercise for about a minute. Now ask yourself whether there is a topic on which you would like to reflect. Do not search too far – simply think of the issue that is currently preoccupying you the most.

Ask yourself:

How does my life situation feel?

Look at the whole picture from a distance without analysing it, as though it were being observed by an onlooker. Create a non-judgemental space and get in touch with the feelings that arise. Now reflect on the qualities that are particularly important to you in your life. If you do not find an answer, simply feel your breath. Now reflect on the matters that have priority in your life. Focus entirely on the first thought that comes to mind. Now direct your attention to your abdominal wall once again and become aware of your breath. Watch the effect of the quality of the breath on your mind. Now move the body according to your current need and end the exercise. This is one of the exercises that I always introduce with great success in my work as a yoga therapist. As Socrates stated – we can always find the important answers within ourselves. It is possible for us to gain deep insights by centring the mind with simple exercises. Many people who have practised this exercise have received important insights and answers to life issues. Others have found it possible to free up repressed, painful feelings and forgive other people, which has helped them to significantly change their lives. Clearly directing the mind towards the qualities that are important at that moment, brings us the clarity to act consciously. It helps us to take the steps required to carry on in life and meet its challenges with joy and trust. Anxiety, uncertainty and worries evaporate into the atmosphere of the wider consciousness.

Self-awareness

Through acceptance and self-reflection, it is possible to look more deeply at ourselves and go into the foundation of the issues we are struggling with. This lets us recognise, for example, the root causes of physical complaints such as back pain. Once we have recognised the unhealthy posture leading to the pain, we will become more aware of our body. Many physical complaints and chronic diseases result from lack of awareness or from reinforcing habits. Well-meaning advice from others is not effective if one's own insight into the problem is missing. It is only by recognising the root cause of our own suffering that we can accept responsibility for our lives and the consequences of our actions. This frees us from the widespread victim mentality and lack of accountability that so many of us project in life. It is very insightful to observe which troubling thoughts and emotions we see again and again leading to this mentality. It is worthwhile to observe how we behave at these times. If we carefully examine our mind, we often succeed in recognising the causes of these painfully recurring thoughts and feelings. Those who immerse themselves in this deep investigation will discover the roots of suffering that inhibit us again and again, namely false understanding, clinging to the ego, aversion, longing and fear. These are the unconscious impulses that confine us time and again.

According to the teachings of Buddha, there are thousands of troubling emotions. Take some time to write down a 'top-ten' list of the ones that trouble you most own. Reflecting on ourselves with deep awareness brings us into contact with the many perceptions and emotions of life. These include pleasant feelings such as satisfaction and serenity and also unpleasant ones such as judgment, dislike, boredom and fear. We constantly experience the fluctuating and persistent nature of these emotions. Powerful feelings such as rage and annoyance affect our entire being through the body, breath and mind. They are stored in the body and leave an impression upon us. As a result, the causes of muscular tension can sometimes be found in suppressed emotions such as illness, rage and old injuries. In my work as physical therapist, I have seen that pressure from only one finger on chronically contracted muscles can release deep feelings and even bring up old trauma. Once these feelings come to the surface, we have the opportunity to consciously experience grief, accept it and to let it go. Allowing the tears to flow requires courage and a safe, familiar environment, can be releasing and liberating. Despite a commonly accepted idea that showing our feelings is an indication of weakness, examining your feelings in this way is a true act of courage. So go head and courageously explore your emotions!

Now, I invite you to try an exercise that will help you identify and understand the roots of strong emotions.

Please read through the exercise first.

1. Take a few deep breaths using the throat-controlled (loud) breathing technique described earlier. Listen to the sound of your breath.

2. Now, relax the throat, and observe a few deep breaths performed without using a particular breathing technique.

3. Notice your body. What do you experience in your body after taking these few breaths?

4. Ask yourself which troubling feelings and thoughts are recurring themes in your life. Become conscious of the causes (roots) of these troubling emotions. Create the space to allow yourself to recognise their roots. Practice taking this awareness into everyday situations and mentally identifying these troubling thoughts and emotions as they arise.

5. If you use this simple awareness practice regularly, you will receive valuable insight into your previously unconscious habits and behaviour. To examine this idea further, you can also ask those close to you about troubling emotions or behaviour that they observe in you. This naturally requires some courage. Now, ask yourself which mental qualities would be helpful for converting troubling feelings into something positive. Give these qualities space to grow in your consciousness.

To conclude the exercise, take a few more deep breaths and relax. In the Yoga Sutras, Patanjali recommends, among other things, four qualities (*Bhavanas*), which we can use to keep our spirits aligned

*   Maitri – kindness.

*   Karuna – compassion.

*   Mudita – vicarious joy.

*   Upeksha – detachment.

By constantly cultivating and internalising these four qualities, we experience a holistic effect and transform our whole being. In the very intensive yoga training courses which last over a month, I am always impressed how effectively these qualities transform people when cultivated regularly. Because of this impressionable experience, I gained an increased sense for appreciation, which I express by telling others about the positive qualities I observe in them. This approach is usually well received, but some find it very challenging, initially, to accept positive feedback.

You can try this technique this very day: say to someone close to you how you value and appreciate them. Observe how this simple action affects both you and your fellow human being.

Self-healing

Yoga practice, with its holistic exercises for the body, breath and mind, offers excellent opportunities for self-healing and transformation. Many physical complaints, such as backache, can be resolved through regular, customised yoga practice. Even chronic conditions, such as high blood pressure and asthma, can be alleviated through yoga, thereby improving the health. The "remedies" of self-acceptance, self-reflection and self-awareness create favourable preconditions for reducing our suffering and living more happily. Support from an experienced yoga therapist can be very helpful in this process. Without the willingness to take responsibility for our own life and regularly practising yoga, we put barriers in the way of sustained and lasting healing. Yoga therapy is primarily about the person and not their complaints or illnesses. Healing occurs when the balance of the inner and outer energies are restored. In this sense, yoga therapy stimulates the self-healing process, in that we ourselves can contribute a great deal to our physical and mental health. Besides its great healing potential, yoga therapy offers us many opportunities to live more consciously and more contentedly.

Transformation through Yoga Meditation

The mental barriers (*kleshas*) and our unconscious tendencies can be reduced and even resolved through regular meditation. Yoga meditation enables us to clear our mind. It opens us up to profound transformation, in which we experience true happiness. In the Yoga Sutras, Patanjali shows us different paths and options for solutions to decrease our suffering, whereby we can effectively alter our mind through meditation techniques. Below, I will introduce you to a meditation technique that is based on the five parts of yoga according to Patanjali. In yoga training courses, I have already taught these techniques successfully for many years. Along with Mantra and Vipassana meditation, I find it the most effective form of meditation. Here we assume a stable sitting position, extend the breath with throat breathing, watch the flow of the breath, focus our mind in becoming aware of the centres of energy (*chakras*) and open our mind to the endless, eternal consciousness of being. The effects of this yoga meditation are:

- Extending the breath

- Increased oxygen intake

- Greater expulsion of carbon dioxide

- Stimulation of the digestive organs

- Strengthening of the lungs and breath volumes

- Alkaline and de-acidifying effect

- Increasing the vital energy and life energy

- Releasing physical and mental tensions

- Physical and mental lightness

- Promoting concentration and alertness

- Mental clarity

- Calming the mind and finding stillness

- Connection with higher wisdom

- Encouraging joy in life and happiness

Instructions for Yoga meditation

Firstly, read the text through carefully.

Stage 1: Stihra Sukhamasanam – stable and pleasant sitting position

Come into a stable and pleasant sitting position on the floor. Use a cushion to support you. If you find it difficult to sit on the floor for 30 minutes, sit on a chair. Assume an upright position and feel the contact with the cushion. Enable yourself to make small adjustments to the position while sitting, should you feel very uncomfortable. However, try to remain as motionless as possible. Try to be patient and limit your movement.

Stage 2: Pranayama – extension of the breath

You should carry out this stage for about 5 minutes. With a gentle sound in the throat (throat breathing) slowly and consciously extend the breath. With this technique you can hear and refine the quality of the breath. Inhale and exhale slowly and regularly. Find a breathing rhythm that suits you. If your thoughts wander, come back to conscious breathing.

Stage 3: Dharana – sustained alignment of the mind

This stage lasts for around 5 minutes. With the next inhalation, feel the sensations at the front of your body Face, throat, chest, abdomen, lower body and pelvic floor.

When you exhale, feel the sensations at the back of your body, from the pelvic floor to the back of the head. For the next inhalation your attention is at the front once again and for the next exhalation it is at the back of the body. Try to be where your breath is flowing at that moment. It is all about your awareness from moment to moment. Always come back to the exercise if your mind or body distract you.

Stage 4: Dhyanam – deep concentration leads to meditation

You should practise this stage for about 12 minutes.

Direct your attention to the highest point in the body, at the cranium of the head. Become aware of your feelings there and watch the flow of energy. Remain with the cranium, forehead area, neck, breastbone and abdomen for about 90 seconds. Then take your attention slowly from the sacrum to the cranium and focus on the sensations on the rear side of your body.

Stage 5: Samyama – immersion via the light at the cranium brings us into the contact with the essence of light

This stage should be carried out for 5 to 10 minutes. Focus your attention on the cranium. Concentrate on the sensations and become aware of the flow of energy. Open your mind to the light at the cranium and immerse yourself in it fully. Become one with the light. Remain in this immersion and always come back when your body or mind is diverted. At the end, come back slowly by taking a few deep breaths. Become aware of the effect of the meditation on your mind, breath and body. Now move your legs slowly and relax the entire body a little. You can practise this form of meditations very well in stages. As a beginner you can start with stages 1-3. Then increase it slowly until you are practising all stages. Do this regularly.

May meditation promote
your health and happiness

Index of the Asanas

Adho Mukha Svanasana (downward facing dog)
Anantasana (snake king pose)
Apanasana (wind-relieving pose)
Ardha Chandrasana (half-moon)
Ardha Dhanurasana (half bow)
Ardha Matsyendrasana (half spinal twist)
Ardha Padma Uttanasana (half bound lotus)
Ardha Parshva Uttanasana (asymmetrical forward bend)
Ardha Shalabhasana (half locust)
Ardha Utkatasana (half chair)
Ardha Uttanasana (standing half forward bend)

Bhagirathasana (tree, also Vrkshasana)
Bharadvajasana (Bharadvaja's twist)
Bhujangasana (cobra)

Catuspadapitham (table top)
Chakravakasana (cat)

Dandasana (staff pose)
Dvipada Pitham (bridge)

Eka Pada Rajakapotasana (pigeon)
Eka Pada Ustrasana (one-legged camel pose)

Gomukhasana (cow's face)

Janu Shirshasana (sitting head to knee pose)
Jathara Parivritti (crocodile)

Kabalabhati (breath lighting the cranium)

Matsyendrasana (spinal twist)

Natarajasana (dancer)
Navasana (boat)

Parshva Konasana (side angle pose)
Parshva Uttanasana (forward bend over one leg)
Paschimottanasana (seated forward bend)

Prasarita Padottanasana (wide-legged forward bend)

Samasthiti (mountain pose)
Shalabhasana (locust)
Shavasana (corpse)
Siddhasana (perfect pose)
Sukhasana (easy pose)
Supta Prasarita Padangusthasana (wide-legged stretch pose)
Supta Baddha Konasana (goddess)

Tadasana (mountain)

Upavista Konasana (wide-angled seated forward bend)
Urdhva Prasarita Padasana (upward stretched legs)
Ustrasana (camel)
Uttanasana (standing forward bend)
Utthita Eka Padangusthasana (standing position with leg stretched forward)
Utthita Trikonasana (extended triangle pose)

Vajrasana (diamond sitting pose)
Vasisthasana (side plank)
Vimanasana (splayed-leg locust)
Vinyasa (flowing sequence of asanas)
Virabhadrasana (hero or warrior pose)

Source references for the anatomy texts

Source references for the anatmoy texts

Klein- Vogelbach, S.: Funktionelle Bewegungslehre (5.Auflage); Bewegung lernen and lehren, Springer Verlag 2000

Mosetter K+ R: Myoreflextherapie, Muskelfunktion und Schmerz, Vesalius Verlag 2001

Dr. med. Ch. Larsen, C. Larsen, O. Hartelt: Körperhaltungen verbessern, Trias Verlag 2008

Meyers Th.: Anatomy Trains, Urban und Fischer Verlag 2004

Lee S-W. et al.: Relationship between low back pain and lumbar multifiduus size at different postures; spine Vol.31 (19) S.2258-2262; 2006

Kapndji I.A.: Funktionelle Anatomie der Gelenke, Bd.3, Enke Verlag 1992).

Lippert H.: Lehrbuch Anatomie, 7. Auflage, Urban u. Fischer Verlag 2006

Kraftsow, Gary: Kraftquelle Yoga Vianova Verlag 2006

Susan Gilbert

Fig. 1. p. 231 (skeleton of the foot)

Fig. 2. p. 231 (foot prints)

Fig. 3. p. 215 (knee axis)

Fig. 5 p. 197 (coxa vara & valga)

Fig. 8. p. 189 (ligaments of pelvis from the dorsal)

Fig. 4. p.110 fig. 1.117 (hip ligaments)

Fig. 6. p.112 fig. 1.120 (abductors)

Fig. 7 p. 111 fig. 1.119 (iliopsoas muscles)

Fig. 9 p. 68 fig. 1.55 (pelvic alignment...)

Figs. 10+15 p. 28 fig. 1.4. (alignment...)

Kraftquelle Yoga; Kraftsow ; Vianova Verlag

Figs. 11+13 p. 156 (axial skeleton)

Fig. 12 p. 207 (pelvis / iliopsoas muscles)

Fig. 14 p. 180 (scoliosis)

Fig. 16 p.28 (diaphragm + retus...)

Fig. 17 p. 179 (chest ...)

Fig. 18 p. 106 (kyphosis)

Fig. 19 p. 163 (dorsal shoulder muscles..)

Fig. 20 p. 164 (dorsal back muscles..)

Contact addresses

The author
Remo Rittiner
Ayur Yoga Center
Remo Rittiner
Chlosstrasse 24
8873 Amden
www.ayuryoga.ch
Tel. 0041 76 565 98 26
Gives training as an Ayur yoga teacher and Ayur yoga therapist around the world

Alexander Hotz and Uta Naumer-Hotz
78467 Döbelstrasse
4D -78462 Constance
uta.naumerhotz@gmail.com
alexander.hotz@gmail.com
Tel. 0049 753 156 707
Practice for myoreflextherapy; hands-on therapy; myoreflexand yoga therapy

Dr. John Switzer
Feldafing
Germany
info@ayurveda-bayern.com
Tel. 0049 8157 7152
Panchakarma therapy

Dr. Chandrakant Pawar
Palus/Maharashtra, India
www.ayurvedavishwa.com
Tel. 00091 98901 680 28
Ayurveda treatment and massage training

Subject Index